The
POTS Syndrome Cookbook

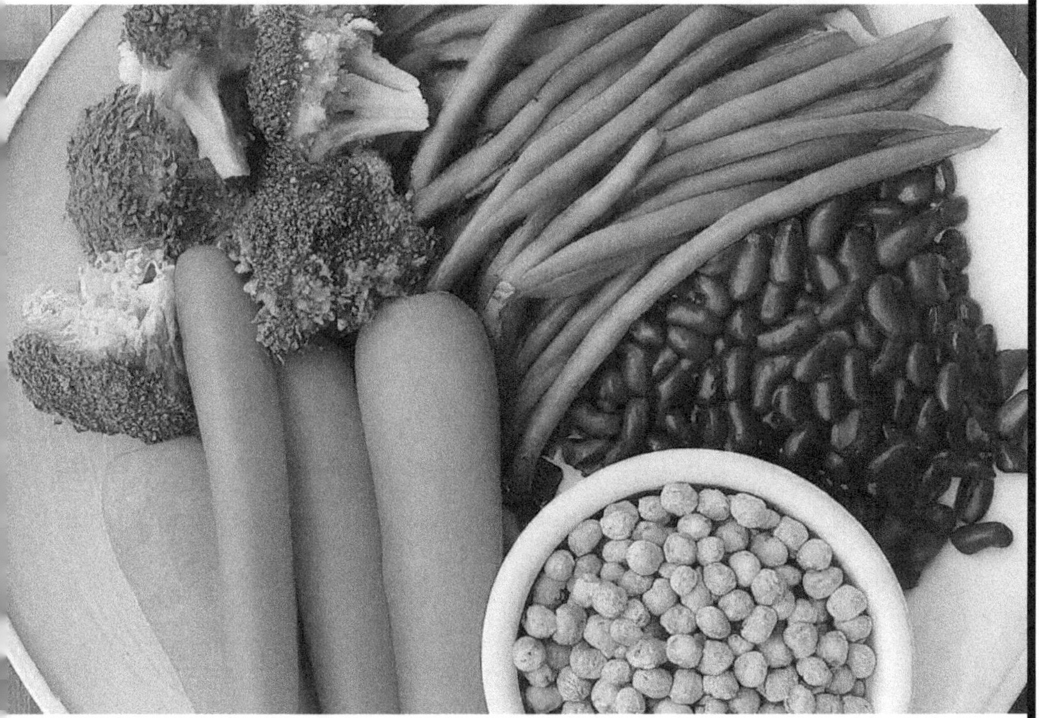

Recipes and Strategies to Increase Energy, Stabilize Blood Pressure, and Reduce Dizziness with High-Salt, Hydrating Foods

Avery Stoneheart

Copyright © 2024 by Avery Stoneheart

All rights reserved. No part of this publication may be reproduced, distributed, or transmitted in any form or by any means, including photocopying, recording, or other electronic or mechanical methods, without the prior written permission of the publisher, except in the case of brief quotations embodied in critical reviews and certain other noncommercial uses permitted by copyright law.

Avery Stoneheart

Contents

Introduction 8
    Fueling Your Body, Managing Your POTS 8
    What is POTS? 9
    The Power of a POTS-Friendly Diet 9

Chapter 1: The Foundations of the POTS Diet 12
    Understanding POTS: A Deeper Look 12
    Decoding the Subtypes 12
    The Pillars of the POTS Diet 14

Chapter 2: Breakfasts to Boost Your Day 18
    Sweet Oats 18
        Tropical Overnight Oats 18
        Pumpkin Spice Power Oats 20
        "PB&B" Bowl 21
    Savory Oats 23
        Savory Spinach & Egg Scramble Oats 23
        Avocado & Everything Oats 24
        Cheesy Mushroom & Quinoa Oats 26
    Smoothies 28

- Green Powerhouse 28
- Tropical Sunshine 30
- Berry Blast 31

Avocado Creations 33
- Avocado Toast Upgrade 33
- Avocado Breakfast Salad 35
- Avocado Stuffed Sweet Potato 37
- Banana "Nice Cream" 39
- Savory Breakfast Bowl 41

Chapter 3: Lunches to Keep You Going 44

Soups 44
- Creamy Roasted Tomato & Lentil Soup 44
- Coconut Curry Butternut Squash Soup 46
- Spicy Chicken & Corn Chowder 48
- Hearty Minestrone 50
- Chilled Cucumber & Avocado Soup 52

Salads 54
- Mediterranean Quinoa Salad 54
- Southwest Black Bean & Avocado Salad 56
- Broccoli & Barley Salad 58
- Asian Noodle Salad 60
- Kale & Lentil Salad 62

Main Dishes 64

Tuna Salad Lettuce Wraps 64

Quinoa Veggie Burgers 68

Shrimp Scampi with Zucchini Noodles 70

Salmon & Roasted Veggie Bowls 72

Chapter 4: Easy and Nourishing Dinners 74

    Flavor-Packed Mains 74

        One-Pan Roasted Chicken & Veggies 74

        Sheet-Pan Salmon with Lemon & Asparagus 76

        Lentil & Mushroom "Shepherd's Pie" 78

        Spicy Shrimp & Quinoa Stir-Fry 80

        Turkey Meatballs with Zucchini Noodles 82

    Light & Refreshing 84

        Mediterranean Chickpea Salad Pitas 84

        Summer Veggie Frittata 86

        Asian-Inspired Lettuce Wraps 88

        Avocado & Black Bean Quesadillas 90

        Tuna Nicoise Salad 92

    Hearty & Comforting 94

        Chicken Pot Pie with Sweet Potato Crust 94

        Slow Cooker Beef Stew 96

        Vegetarian Chili 98

        Lentil & Butternut Squash "Lasagna" 100

        Stuffed Acorn Squash 102

Chapter 5: Snacks, Sips, and Smart Choices 104

Savory Snacks 104

- Salty Trail Mix 104
- Pickle Roll-Ups 106
- Crunchy Corned Beef Bites 108
- Savory Yogurt Dip 109

Hydrating & Refreshing 112

- Fruit & Veggie Skewers 112
- Chia Seed Pudding 113
- Frozen Grapes 114
- Banana "Nice Cream" 115
- Avocado Smoothie 116
- Electrolyte Popsicles 117
- Fruit-Infused Water 118
- Herbal Iced Tea 119

Chapter 6: Living Well with POTS 120

Beyond the Plate: Lifestyle Factors 120

- Exercise: 120
- Stress Management: 121
- Sleep Tips: 121
- The Importance of Individualization 122

Success Story: Alex's Journey 123

Appendix 125

7-day meal plan 125

Food Conversion Charts (Sodium content, etc.) 127

Why Use Them for POTS Management? 128

How to Use Food Conversion Charts 128

28 DAYS MEAL PLANNER TEMPLATE & SHOPPING LIST
.... 131

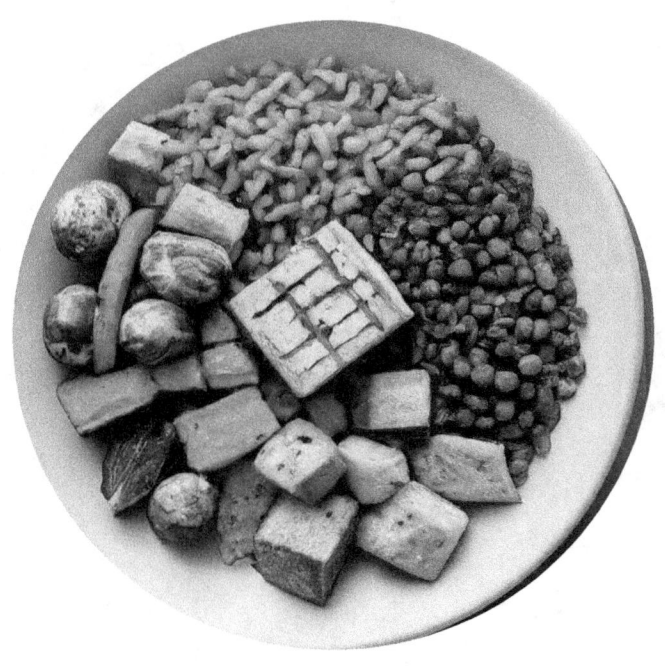

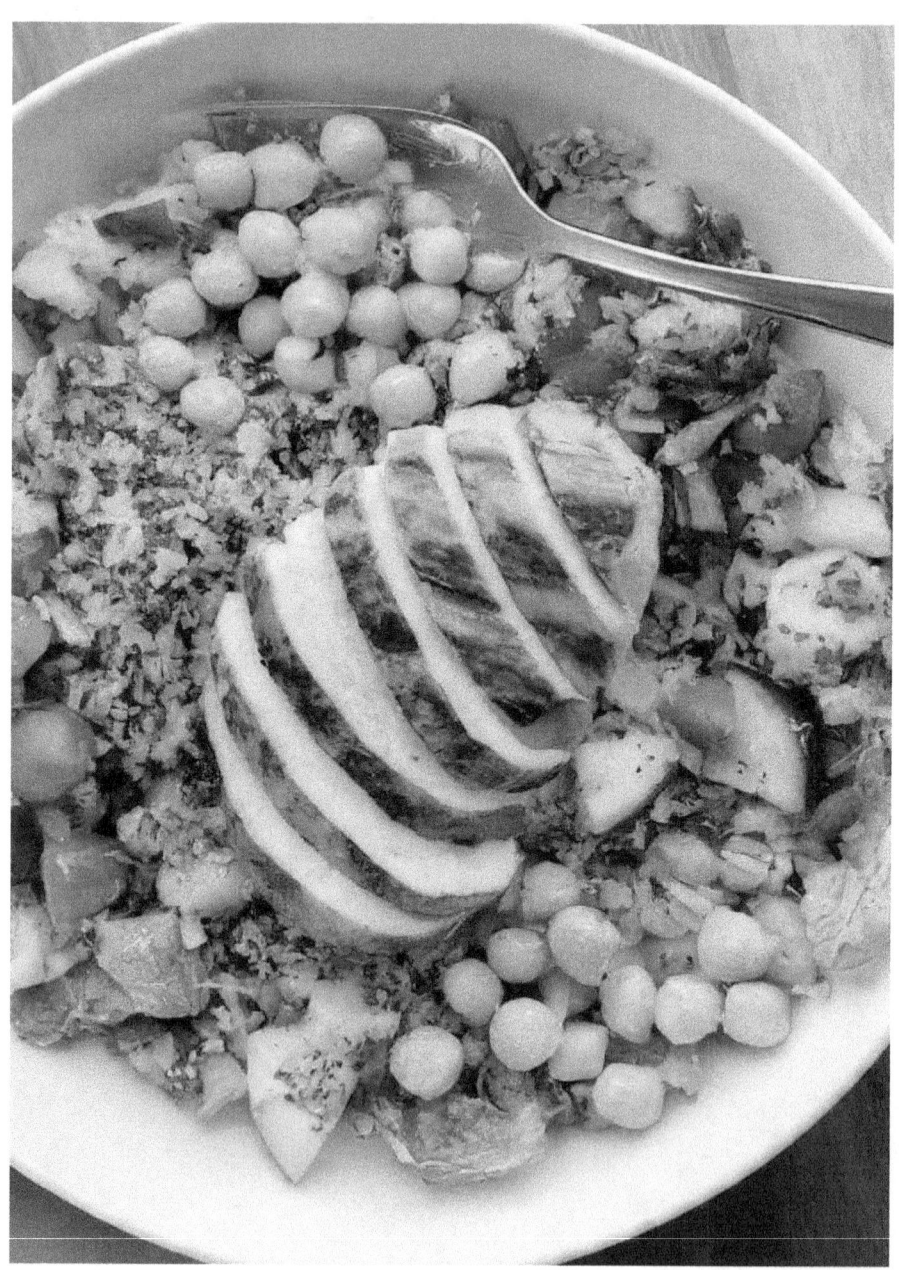

Introduction

Fueling Your Body, Managing Your POTS

Welcome to a world of flavorful food that can make a profound difference in your life. If you're living with Postural Orthostatic Tachycardia Syndrome (POTS), you know the challenges it presents: the dizziness, the fatigue, the racing heart, and the feeling that your body is working against you.

But what if I told you that what's on your plate could be a powerful tool in managing your POTS symptoms?

I'm Avery Stoneheart, a nutritionist specializing in POTS, and I understand both the science behind this condition and the everyday struggles it creates. After years of research, recipe development, and working with countless POTS patients, I've seen firsthand how the right diet can improve energy levels, reduce dizziness, and enhance your overall quality of life.

Whether you're newly diagnosed, or you've been managing POTS for years, this cookbook is your key to reclaiming control of your health.

What is POTS?

Let's start with a quick overview of POTS. Simply put, it's a dysfunction of the autonomic nervous system – the part of your body that controls automatic functions like heart rate, blood pressure, and digestion. ***POTS can cause a constellation of symptoms, including:***

1. Dizziness and lightheadedness, especially upon standing
2. Rapid heartbeat (tachycardia)
3. Fatigue and weakness
4. Brain fog
5. Digestive issues
6. And more...

POTS can be further grouped into different subtypes (hyperadrenergic, neuropathic, hypovolemic) which your doctor can help you understand.

The Power of a POTS-Friendly Diet

While there's no one-size-fits-all cure for POTS, dietary changes can make a significant impact. This cookbook focuses on:

1. **Sodium:** The cornerstone of POTS nutrition, increasing salt intake helps maintain blood volume and reduce symptoms.
2. **Hydration:** Staying hydrated with fluids and electrolytes is crucial.

3. **Nutrient Balance:** Whole foods provide the vitamins and minerals your body needs to function optimally.

This cookbook isn't just about what to eat – it's about enjoying food again. You'll find delicious recipes, practical tips, and the guidance you need to make nourishing meals tailored to your POTS journey.

Let's get started!

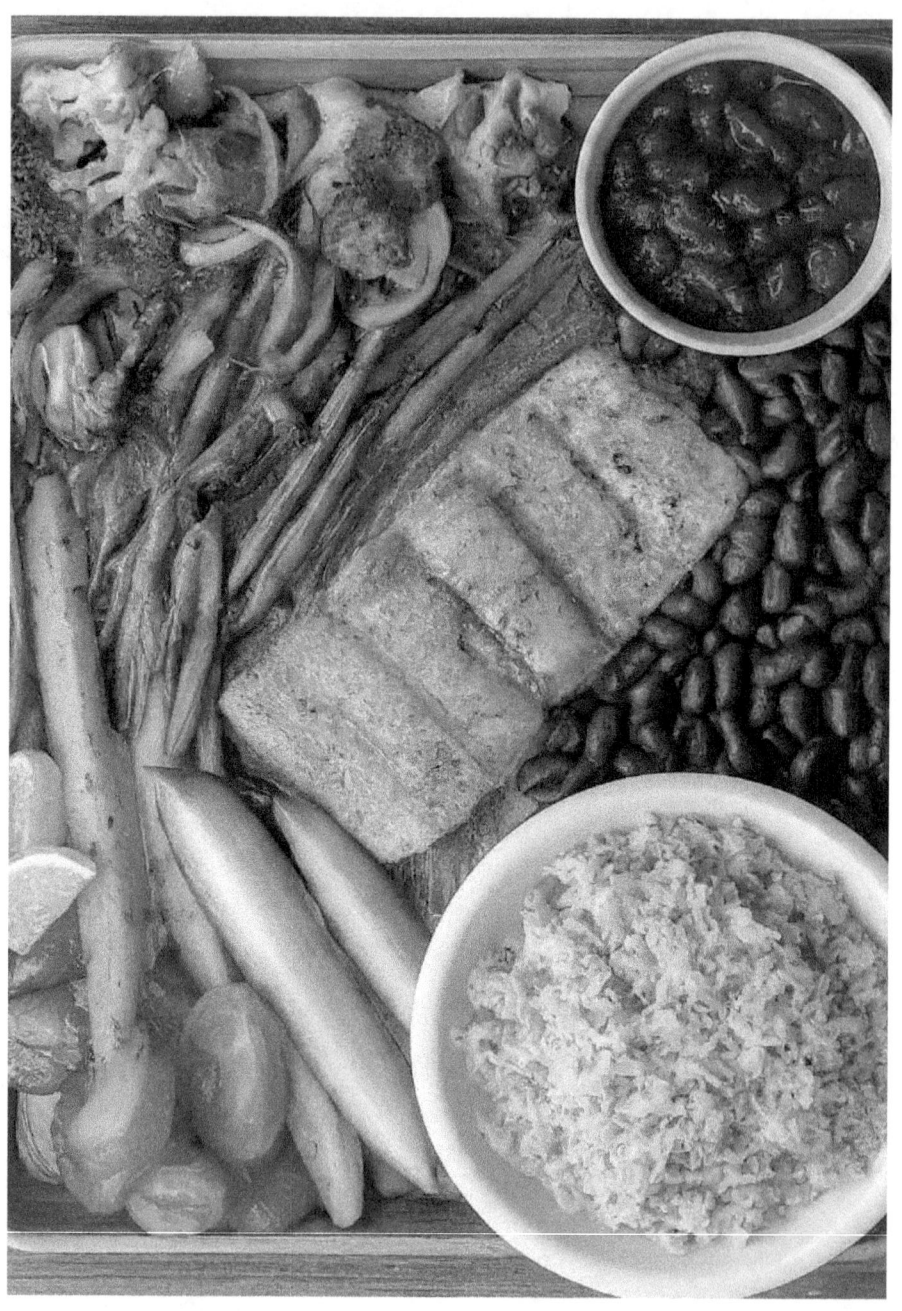

Chapter 1: The Foundations of the POTS Diet

Understanding POTS: A Deeper Look

In the introduction, we touched on the basics of POTS. Now, let's dive deeper so you can better understand how your specific symptoms relate to your dietary needs.

POTS Isn't One-Size-Fits-All: Everyone experiences POTS a little differently. Some people feel faint after a short time standing, others struggle with severe fatigue, and some even notice their legs turning a purplish color. These variations give us clues about which type of POTS you might have.

Decoding the Subtypes

The most common subtypes of POTS are:

1. **Hypovolemic POTS:** Think of this like having a smaller "gas tank." Your blood volume is lower, making you more sensitive to dehydration. Boosting salt and fluids is extra important for you.
2. **Neuropathic POTS:** The tiny nerves in your legs that control blood flow aren't working as well as they should.

Compression stockings can help, along with a focus on the POTS diet basics.

3. **Hyperadrenergic POTS:** Your body is pumping out too much adrenaline – it's like being on a rollercoaster all the time. Cutting back on caffeine and managing stress can complement your diet changes.

Beyond the Basics

1. **Sometimes, There's More:** POTS can sometimes develop because of another medical condition – this is called secondary POTS.
2. **Kids Get It Too:** While POTS in teens often improves on its own, a supportive diet during those years is super important.
3. **It's Not Just About Food:** Understanding what triggers your POTS flare-ups (like hot weather or standing for too long) helps you manage your symptoms overall.

Why This Matters

Knowing your POTS subtype isn't just about labeling it. It helps you and your doctor create the best treatment plan. And that personalized plan will include the perfect diet adjustments for YOU!

A Patient's Story

One of my patients, a young woman who battled constant dizziness, fatigue, and a racing heart, initially thought she was simply out of shape. After finally receiving a diagnosis, she discovered the root of her problems: hyperadrenergic POTS. All that caffeine she relied on to boost her energy was actually making her symptoms worse! By switching to decaf, managing her condition with medication, and adopting a POTS-friendly diet, she experienced a dramatic improvement in her quality of life.

The Pillars of the POTS Diet

Managing POTS isn't just about what you eat; it's about a strategic approach to nutrition. Let's break down the essential pillars of a POTS-friendly diet:

Salt: Your New Best Friend

1. **Why Is It Crucial?** People with POTS often have lower blood volume, and salt helps your body retain more fluid. This increases blood volume and helps prevent those frustrating drops in blood pressure that cause dizziness, fatigue, and other symptoms.
2. **How Much Is Enough?** While the average person is advised to limit sodium, those with POTS usually need much more –

think 3-5 grams of sodium per day, or even higher for some. Don't worry, we'll cover delicious ways to reach those goals! Always consult with your doctor to personalize your salt intake.

3. **Flavorful Salt Boosters:** Get creative with salty favorites like olives, pickles, cured meats, cheeses, miso paste, and soy sauce. Many flavorful condiments are naturally high in salt. We'll explore tasty and satisfying ways to add them to your meals!

Hydration is Key

1. **Fluids Beyond Water:** While water is essential, it may not be enough for POTS. Electrolyte-rich options like broths, coconut water, herbal teas, and even fruits like watermelon provide extra hydration and minerals that your body needs.
2. **Smart Hydration Strategies:** Don't chug it all at once! Sip consistently throughout the day, use a marked water bottle to track intake, and set reminders on your phone.
3. **Signs of Dehydration:** Even mild dehydration worsens POTS. Watch for dark urine, thirst, headaches, and fatigue. If these appear, it's time to boost your fluids!

Electrolyte Essentials

1. **The Big Three:** Sodium, potassium, and magnesium are your electrolyte superstars. Sodium we've covered, but potassium and magnesium are also vital for nerve function, muscle contraction, and keeping your body's fluid balance in check.
2. **Food Sources:** Potassium powerhouses include bananas, avocados, leafy greens, sweet potatoes, and beans. Magnesium stars are nuts, seeds, dark chocolate, and (bonus!) those same leafy greens. Good thing high-salt foods often cover sodium!
3. **Supplements Under Guidance:** Electrolyte drinks, powders, and supplements exist, but always talk to your doctor first. Getting electrolytes through food is often ideal, but sometimes supplementation is helpful.

Beyond the Basics: Nutrients for POTS

1. **Vitamins and Minerals:** Your body runs on various nutrients. B vitamins, iron, and vitamin D play key roles in energy production, blood health, and overall well-being. Deficiencies are common and can worsen POTS symptoms.
2. **Whole Foods Focus:** The best way to get these nutrients is through a diverse diet packed with colorful fruits,

vegetables, whole grains, legumes, nuts, seeds, and lean proteins. Don't worry, delicious doesn't have to mean boring!

These pillars form the foundation of a POTS-friendly way of eating. In the upcoming chapters, we'll dive deeper, with recipes, tips, and strategies to make these principles work for you — deliciously!

Chapter 2: Breakfasts to Boost Your Day

Sweet Oats

Tropical Overnight Oats

- **POTS Power:** Coconut milk provides healthy fats and electrolytes, while mango and banana deliver potassium. Chia seeds add fiber and a little extra protein.
- **Breakfast Boost:** Preparing these the night before streamlines your morning, making them perfect for busy days.

Ingredients:

- 1/2 cup rolled oats
- 1/2 cup coconut milk (unsweetened)
- 1/4 cup diced mango
- 1/4 cup sliced banana
- 1 tablespoon chia seeds
- Pinch of cinnamon (optional)

Instructions
1. Combine all ingredients in a glass jar or container with a lid.
2. Stir well, cover, and refrigerate overnight (or at least 4 hours).
3. Enjoy cold or gently warmed.

Prep Time: 5 minutes
Cook Time: None (overnight soak)
Nutritional Info (approx. per serving):
- Calories: 350,
- Sodium: 80mg,
- Potassium: 500mg,
- Fiber: 10g

Tips: Top with extra fruit, a drizzle of honey, or a sprinkle of toasted coconut for variation.

Pumpkin Spice Power Oats

- **POTS Power:** Pumpkin is packed with potassium, fiber, and antioxidants. Warming spices like cinnamon and nutmeg boost flavor and have anti-inflammatory properties. Walnuts add healthy fats and a touch of protein.
- **Breakfast Boost:** This cozy oatmeal is perfect for fall or whenever you crave a comforting, nutrient-rich breakfast.

Ingredients:

- 1/2 cup rolled oats
- 1 cup milk of choice (almond, soy, etc.)
- 1/4 cup pumpkin puree (canned or homemade)
- 1 tablespoon maple syrup (or sweetener of choice)
- 1/2 teaspoon pumpkin pie spice
- Pinch of salt
- 1/4 cup chopped walnuts

Instructions:

1. Combine oats, milk, pumpkin puree, maple syrup, pumpkin pie spice, and salt in a small saucepan.
2. Bring to a simmer over medium heat, stirring occasionally. Cook for 5-7 minutes, or until oats are thickened.
3. Stir in chopped walnuts and serve warm.

Prep Time: 5 minutes **Cook Time:** 5-7 minutes

Nutritional Info (approx. per serving): Calories: 380, Sodium: 120mg, Potassium: 450mg, Fiber: 8g

Tips: Top with a dollop of yogurt, an extra sprinkle of pumpkin pie spice, or a drizzle of honey for added sweetness.

"PB&B" Bowl

- **POTS Power:** Peanut butter is a good source of protein, healthy fats, and potassium. Banana adds additional potassium and sweetness. Hemp seeds provide a boost of fiber, iron, and omega-3 fatty acids.
- **Breakfast Boost:** This simple and satisfying bowl keeps you energized all morning and offers a delicious way to get extra nutrients.

Ingredients:

- 1/2 cup rolled oats
- 1 cup milk of choice (almond, soy, etc.)
- 1 tablespoon creamy peanut butter
- 1/2 banana, sliced
- 1 tablespoon hemp seeds
- Pinch of cinnamon (optional)

Instructions:

1. Combine oats and milk in a saucepan. Bring to a simmer over medium heat, stirring occasionally. Cook for 5-7 minutes, or until oats are thickened.
2. Remove from heat and stir in peanut butter until smooth.
3. Transfer oatmeal to a bowl and top with sliced banana, hemp seeds, and a sprinkle of cinnamon (if desired).

Prep Time: 5 minutes

Cook Time: 5-7 minutes

Nutritional Info (approx. per serving):

- Calories: 400,
- Sodium: 150mg,
- Potassium: 550mg,
- Fiber: 9g

Tips: Use other nut butters (almond, cashew) or seed butters (sunflower) for variation. Add a drizzle of honey or maple syrup for a touch of extra sweetness.

Savory Oats

Savory Spinach & Egg Scramble Oats

- **POTS Power:** Eggs add protein, spinach provides iron and potassium, the broth base boosts hydration and sodium.
- **Breakfast Boost:** A hearty and satisfying option to keep you fueled all morning.

Ingredients:

- 1/2 cup rolled oats
- 1 cup vegetable or chicken broth
- 1/2 cup baby spinach
- 1 egg
- 1 tablespoon olive oil
- Pinch of salt, pepper, and hot sauce (optional)

Instructions

1. Heat olive oil in a pan, add spinach and saute until wilted. Remove and set aside.
2. In the same pan, whisk the egg. Scramble until cooked through.
3. In a separate pot, bring broth to a simmer and add oats. Cook as per package directions.
4. Stir in cooked spinach and scrambled egg. Season to taste.

Prep Time: 5 minutes **Cook Time:** 10-12 minutes

Nutritional Info (approx. per serving): Calories: 300, Sodium: 450mg, Potassium: 600mg, Protein: 15g

Tips: Top with a dollop of plain yogurt, avocado slices, or your favorite hot sauce.

Avocado & Everything Oats

- **POTS Power:** Avocado offers healthy fats, fiber, and a good dose of potassium. "Everything bagel" seasoning adds a burst of flavor and a sodium boost. The poached egg provides protein and additional nutrients.
- **Breakfast Boost:** This savory and satisfying dish offers a delicious way to incorporate more salt and healthy fats into your morning routine.

Ingredients:

- 1/2 cup rolled oats
- 1 cup vegetable or chicken broth
- 1/4 avocado, mashed
- 1 poached egg
- 1 tablespoon "everything bagel" seasoning
- Pinch of salt, pepper (optional)

Instructions:

1. Bring broth to a simmer in a small saucepan and add oats. Cook as per package directions.
2. While the oats cook, poach your egg. (There are many methods - find one that works best for you!)
3. Once cooked, stir the mashed avocado into the oats until creamy. Season with a pinch of salt and pepper if desired.
4. Transfer oats to a bowl. Top with the poached egg and a generous sprinkle of "everything bagel" seasoning.

Prep Time: 5 minutes

Cook Time: 10-12 minutes (including poaching the egg)

Nutritional Info (approx. per serving):

- Calories: 400,
- Sodium: 550mg,
- Potassium: 700mg,
- Fiber: 9g,
- Protein: 18g

Tips:

- For extra flavor, saute a bit of chopped onion or garlic with the oats before adding the broth.
- Top with sliced cherry tomatoes or a sprinkle of fresh herbs for a pop of color and freshness.
- Don't like poached eggs? Substitute a fried or scrambled egg instead.

Cheesy Mushroom & Quinoa Oats

- **POTS Power:** Combining oats and quinoa creates a complete protein, while mushrooms offer earthy flavor and additional nutrients. Parmesan provides a salty kick and a touch of calcium.
- **Breakfast Boost:** This hearty and satisfying dish delivers sustained energy and plenty of flavorful complexity for a change of pace.

Ingredients:

- 1/4 cup quinoa
- 1/4 cup rolled oats
- 1 cup vegetable or chicken broth
- 1/2 cup sliced mushrooms
- 1 tablespoon olive oil
- 1 tablespoon grated Parmesan cheese
- Fresh herbs for garnish (parsley, basil, chives), optional
- Pinch of salt and pepper

Instructions:

1. Rinse quinoa thoroughly. Combine quinoa, oats, and broth in a small saucepan. Bring to a simmer and cook for 15-20 minutes, or until liquid is absorbed.
2. While the grains cook, heat olive oil in a pan. Sauté mushrooms until softened and slightly browned.

3. Stir the cooked mushrooms and Parmesan cheese into the oats and quinoa mixture. Season with salt and pepper to taste.
4. Garnish with fresh herbs (if using) and enjoy warm.

Prep Time: 5 minutes

Cook Time: 20-25 minutes

Nutritional Info (approx. per serving):

- Calories: 350,
- Sodium: 500mg,
- Potassium: 450mg, Fiber: 7g,
- Protein: 15g

Tips:

- Use your favorite variety of mushrooms (cremini, shiitake, etc.)
- For extra creaminess, stir in a dollop of ricotta or a splash of milk at the end.
- Add a pinch of red pepper flakes for a bit of heat.

Smoothies

Green Powerhouse

- **POTS Power:** Spinach is packed with potassium, antioxidants, and fiber. Banana adds potassium and sweetness, while almond butter delivers healthy fats and protein. Protein powder provides an extra nutritional boost.
- **Smoothie Success:** Perfect for on-the-go mornings when you need a quick and energizing breakfast option.

Ingredients:

- 1 cup packed baby spinach
- 1 frozen banana
- 1 tablespoon almond butter
- 1 scoop protein powder (vanilla or unflavored)
- 1 cup almond milk (or your preferred milk)
- Handful of ice (optional, for a thicker smoothie)

Instructions:

1. Add all ingredients to a high-powered blender.
2. Blend until smooth and creamy. Add more liquid if needed to reach desired consistency.

Prep Time: 5 minutes

Blend Time: 1-2 minutes

Nutritional Info (approx. per serving):

- Calories: 350,
- Sodium: 150mg,
- Potassium: 800mg,
- Fiber: 10g,
- Protein: 25g

Tips:

- Use ripe or frozen bananas for optimal sweetness.
- Choose protein powder that fits your dietary needs and taste preferences.
- Add a tablespoon of chia seeds or flaxseeds for extra fiber and healthy fats.

Tropical Sunshine

- **POTS Power:** Mango and pineapple are loaded with potassium and vitamin C. Coconut milk contributes electrolytes and healthy fats. Greek yogurt adds protein and a creamy texture.
- **Smoothie Success:** This tropical treat delivers a burst of sunshine and nutrients, perfect for a refreshing breakfast or a post-workout pick-me-up.

Ingredients:

- 1 cup frozen mango chunks
- 1 cup frozen pineapple chunks
- 1/2 cup coconut milk (unsweetened)
- 1/2 cup Greek yogurt (plain)
- Squeeze of lime juice (optional)

Instructions:

1. Combine all ingredients in a blender.
2. Blend until smooth, adding a splash of water if needed for consistency.

Prep Time: 5 minutes **Blend Time:** 1-2 minutes

Nutritional Info (approx. per serving): Calories: 300, Sodium: 100mg, Potassium: 650mg, Fiber: 7g, Protein: 12g

Tips:

- Use fresh mango and pineapple if in season.
- Top with a sprinkle of shredded coconut for a tropical touch.

Berry Blast

- **POTS Power:** Berries are rich in potassium, antioxidants and fiber. Avocado boosts healthy fats and potassium, while chia seeds offer fiber, omega-3 fatty acids, and a touch of protein.
- **Smoothie Success:** This smoothie offers a delicious combination of sweetness, tartness, and creamy texture. It's great for a refreshing breakfast or a healthy snack.

Ingredients:

- 1 cup mixed frozen berries (blueberries, raspberries, strawberries, etc.)
- 1/2 avocado
- 1 tablespoon chia seeds
- 1 cup oat milk (or your preferred milk)
- 1 teaspoon honey (or sweetener of choice)
- Handful of ice (optional)

Instructions:

1. Add all ingredients to a high-powered blender.
2. Blend until completely smooth and creamy. Add more oat milk if needed to achieve desired consistency.

Prep Time: 5 minutes **Blend Time:** 1-2 minutes

Nutritional Info (approx. per serving):

- Calories: 320,
- Sodium: 90mg,
- Potassium: 600mg,
- Fiber: 12g,
- Protein: 8g

Tips:

- Use a mix of your favorite berries for a vibrant flavor.
- Adjust the honey/sweetener to your desired level of sweetness.
- For extra protein, add a scoop of your preferred protein powder.

Avocado Creations

Avocado Toast Upgrade

- **POTS Power:** Avocado delivers healthy fats, fiber, and potassium. Whole grain toast offers complex carbohydrates for sustained energy. The addition of a fried egg provides protein, while tomatoes and pumpkin seeds add flavor, nutrients, and a satisfying salt boost.
- **Breakfast Boost:** This classic gets revamped for POTS needs. It's customizable and delicious.

Ingredients:

- 1 slice whole-grain bread
- 1/2 avocado, mashed
- 1 fried egg
- 2-3 cherry tomatoes, sliced
- 1 tablespoon pumpkin seeds
- Pinch of salt, pepper, or other spices to taste

Instructions:

1. Toast bread to your desired crispness.
2. Spread mashed avocado on toast.
3. Top with fried egg, sliced tomatoes, and a sprinkle of pumpkin seeds.
4. Season with salt, pepper, and spices like red pepper flakes or paprika if desired.

Prep Time: 5 minutes **Cook Time:** 5 minutes (for the fried egg)

Nutritional Info (approx. per serving): Calories: 450, Sodium: 400mg, Potassium: 800mg, Fiber: 12g, Protein: 20g

Tips:

- Choose a whole-grain bread with a good amount of sodium per slice.
- Use your favorite method to cook the egg.

Avocado Breakfast Salad

- **POTS Power:** This salad is packed with colorful veggies, boosting potassium and overall nutrient intake. Cucumber and red onion add freshness, feta cheese provides saltiness, and almonds offer healthy fats and a satisfying crunch.
- **Breakfast Boost:** A light and refreshing option, perfect for warmer days or when you want a break from heavier meals.

Ingredients:

- 1 avocado, diced
- 1/2 cucumber, diced
- 1/4 cup diced red onion
- 1/4 cup crumbled feta cheese
- 1 tablespoon chopped almonds
- Lemon vinaigrette (recipe below)

Lemon Vinaigrette:

- 2 tablespoons olive oil
- 1 tablespoon lemon juice
- Pinch of salt, pepper, dried herbs (like oregano or dill)

Instructions:

1. Combine all salad ingredients (avocado, cucumber, red onion, feta, almonds) in a bowl.
2. Make the vinaigrette: Whisk together olive oil, lemon juice, salt, pepper, and dried herbs.
3. Drizzle the vinaigrette over the salad and toss to coat.

Prep Time: 10 minutes

Nutritional Info (approx. per serving):

- Calories: 380,
- Sodium: 350mg,
- Potassium: 650mg,
- Fiber: 9g,
- Protein: 12g

Tips:

- Add other POTS-friendly chopped vegetables like bell peppers, olives, or tomatoes.
- Top with a grilled chicken breast for extra protein.

Avocado Stuffed Sweet Potato

- **POTS Power:** Sweet potatoes are rich in potassium, fiber, and vitamin A. Avocado adds healthy fats and additional potassium. Black beans provide protein and fiber, while salsa adds flavor and some extra veggies.
- **Breakfast Boost:** This dish offers a balance of complex carbs, healthy fats, and protein for sustained energy. It's a warm and comforting option for cooler mornings.

Ingredients:

- 1 medium sweet potato
- 1/2 avocado, mashed
- 1/4 cup black beans (canned or cooked)
- 1/4 cup salsa
- 1 tablespoon sour cream (or plain Greek yogurt)
- Pinch of salt, pepper, chili powder, or other spices to taste

Instructions:

1. **Bake the Sweet Potato:** Pierce sweet potato with a fork and bake at 400°F (200°C) for 45-60 minutes, or until tender. (Can also be microwaved for a quicker option).
2. **Prep the Fillings:** While the sweet potato bakes, rinse black beans if using canned. Prepare your salsa and spices.
3. **Assemble:** Once baked, slice the sweet potato lengthwise and gently fluff the insides with a fork.

4. **Fill:** Mash avocado and spread inside the sweet potato. Top with black beans, salsa, and a dollop of sour cream or yogurt. Season with salt, pepper, and spices to your liking.

Prep Time: 10 minutes **Cook Time:** 45-60 minutes (mostly for the sweet potato)

Nutritional Info (approx. per serving):

- Calories: 450,
- Sodium: 300mg,
- Potassium: 1200mg,
- Fiber: 15g,
- Protein: 15g

Tips:

- For extra spice, add a drizzle of hot sauce or a sprinkle of cayenne pepper.
- Top with crumbled feta cheese for extra saltiness and flavor.
- Use leftover baked sweet potatoes to make this dish even faster.

Banana "Nice Cream"

- **POTS Power:** Bananas are a potassium powerhouse. This simple recipe lets you enjoy a creamy, frozen treat without added sugar while getting in those essential electrolytes.
- **Nice Cream Know-How:** The key is using very ripe bananas, ideally ones with plenty of brown spots. Frozen in chunks, they blend into a surprisingly ice-cream-like texture.

Ingredients (for a basic recipe):

- 2-3 frozen bananas, cut into chunks
- Splash of milk (almond, soy, etc.), optional

Instructions:

1. Add frozen banana chunks to a food processor or high-powered blender.
2. Blend until completely smooth and creamy. A splash of milk can help if it seems too thick.
3. Serve immediately for a soft-serve consistency, or freeze for a firmer scoopable texture.

Topping Ideas:

- Fresh berries (raspberries, blueberries, sliced strawberries)
- Cacao nibs for a touch of chocolatey crunch
- Chopped nuts (almonds, pecans)
- Drizzle of nut butter
- Sprinkle of granola

Electrolyte Popsicles
- **POTS Power:** Watermelon and cucumber are highly hydrating, and both offer some potassium. The addition of a pinch of salt provides sodium, and electrolyte powder (if used) boosts other essential minerals.
- **Popsicle Perfection:** These refreshing popsicles are great for hot days or when you need an extra hydration and electrolyte boost.

Ingredients:
- 2 cups cubed watermelon
- 1/2 cup diced cucumber
- Pinch of salt
- Squeeze of lime juice
- 1 scoop electrolyte powder (optional)

Instructions:
1. Combine all ingredients in a blender. Blend until completely smooth.
2. Pour mixture into popsicle molds and freeze for at least 4 hours, or until solid.

Tips:
- Get creative with the flavors! Add a small handful of mint or basil leaves before blending for a fresh twist.
- If you don't have popsicle molds, use small paper cups and popsicle sticks.

Savory Breakfast Bowl

- **POTS Power**: This bowl delivers a powerhouse of nutrients and electrolytes. Quinoa and brown rice provide complex carbs and protein, veggies offer potassium and fiber, Greek yogurt and feta boost saltiness, and almonds add healthy fats and crunch.

- **Breakfast Boost:** A warm and satisfying option, customizable to your preferences and packed with the nutrients you need to start your day.

Ingredients:

Base:

- 1/2 cup cooked quinoa
- 1/2 cup cooked brown rice

Veggies:

- 1/2 cup diced sweet potato
- 1/4 cup diced red bell pepper
- 1/2 cup baby spinach
- 1 tablespoon olive oil

Flavor Boost:

- 1/2 teaspoon cumin
- 1/4 teaspoon paprika
- Pinch of salt and pepper

- Squeeze of lemon juice
- Handful of fresh cilantro or parsley, chopped

Toppings:
- 2 tablespoons Greek yogurt
- 2 tablespoons crumbled feta cheese
- 1 tablespoon toasted almonds

Instructions:
1. Cook the Base: If not already prepared, cook quinoa and brown rice according to package instructions.
2. Sauté the Veggies: Heat olive oil in a pan. Add sweet potato and cook until slightly softened. Add bell pepper and spinach, sauté until spinach is wilted.
3. Season: Stir in cumin, paprika, salt, and pepper. Finish with a squeeze of lemon juice.
4. Assemble: Combine cooked quinoa and brown rice in a bowl. Top with the sautéed veggie mixture.
5. Add Toppings: Dollop with Greek yogurt, sprinkle with feta cheese and toasted almonds. Garnish with fresh herbs.

Prep Time: 10 minutes **Cook Time**: 15-20 minutes (depending on if rice and quinoa are pre-cooked)

Nutritional Info (approx. per serving):

- Calories: 500,
- Sodium: 550mg,
- Potassium: 900mg,
- Fiber: 12g,
- Protein: 20g

Tips:

- Get Creative with Veggies: Add other POTS-friendly vegetables like broccoli, zucchini, or mushrooms.
- Change the Spices: Use your favorite spice blends for different flavor profiles.
- Make it Ahead: Prep the base and veggies in advance for a quick assembly in the morning.

Chapter 3: Lunches to Keep You Going

Soups

Creamy Roasted Tomato & Lentil Soup

- **POTS Power:** Roasted tomatoes offer concentrated flavor and potassium. Lentils boost protein and fiber, while a touch of cream adds richness, which can also help fats and fat-soluble vitamins be absorbed.
- **Lunchtime Love:** This soup is hearty enough to be a satisfying meal, especially when paired with a slice of whole-grain bread or crackers for dipping.

Ingredients

- 2 tablespoons olive oil
- 1 onion, chopped
- 2 cloves garlic, minced
- 1 (28-ounce) can roasted tomatoes
- 1 cup red lentils
- 4 cups vegetable broth
- 1/4 cup heavy cream (or full-fat coconut milk)
- Salt, pepper, dried herbs (basil, oregano) to taste
- Crumbled feta and fresh basil for garnish

Instructions

1. Heat olive oil in a large pot. Saute onion until softened. Add garlic and cook for another minute.
2. Stir in roasted tomatoes, lentils, broth, and bring to a simmer. Cook covered for 20-25 minutes, or until lentils are tender.
3. Blend soup until smooth (immersion blender or regular blender). Stir in cream, season with salt, pepper, and herbs.
4. Garnish with crumbled feta and fresh basil before serving.

Prep Time: 10 minutes **Cook Time:** 30-35 minutes

Nutritional Info (approx. per serving):

- Calories: 300,
- Sodium: 450mg,
- Potassium: 700mg,
- Fiber: 12g
- , Protein: 15g

Tips:

- Roast your own tomatoes for maximum flavor.
- Add other POTS-friendly veggies like carrots or celery.
- Use a squeeze of lemon juice to brighten the flavor.

Coconut Curry Butternut Squash Soup

- **POTS Power:** Butternut squash is high in potassium and fiber. Coconut milk adds creaminess and healthy fats. Warming curry spices are anti-inflammatory and add flavor complexity.
- **Lunchtime Love:** This soup is comforting and satisfying, with a touch of exotic flavor. Perfect for fall or winter days.

Ingredients:

- 1 tablespoon olive oil
- 1 onion, chopped
- 2 cloves garlic, minced
- 2 pounds butternut squash, peeled, seeded, and cubed
- 1 (14-ounce) can chickpeas, rinsed and drained
- 1 (14-ounce) can full-fat coconut milk
- 4 cups vegetable broth
- 1 tablespoon curry powder
- Salt, pepper to taste
- Chopped cilantro and roasted pumpkin seeds for garnish

Instructions:

1. Heat olive oil in a pot. Sauté onion and garlic until softened.
2. Add butternut squash, chickpeas, coconut milk, broth, and curry powder. Bring to a simmer, then cook covered for 20-25 minutes, or until squash is tender.
3. Blend soup until smooth. Season with salt and pepper.

4. Top with cilantro and roasted pumpkin seeds before serving.

Prep Time: 15 minutes **Cook Time:** 30-35 minutes

Nutritional Info (approx. per serving):

- Calories: 350,
- Sodium: 350mg,
- Potassium: 900mg,
- Fiber: 10g,
- Protein: 10g

Tips:

- Use another type of winter squash (acorn, kabocha) for variation.
- Adjust the level of curry powder to your preferred spice level.
- Add a squeeze of lime juice for a hint of freshness.

Spicy Chicken & Corn Chowder

- **POTS Power:** Chicken provides protein, corn adds sweetness and fiber, while potatoes contribute complex carbs and potassium. The creamy broth offers fats, and the touch of spice can stimulate the appetite.
- **Lunchtime Love:** This chowder is hearty and satisfying, with a bit of a kick for those who enjoy spice. Serve it with a dollop of sour cream for extra richness and saltiness.

Ingredients:

- 1 tablespoon olive oil
- 1 onion, chopped
- 2 celery stalks, chopped
- 1 pound boneless, skinless chicken breast, cut into bite-sized pieces
- 1 teaspoon smoked paprika
- 1/2 teaspoon chili powder (adjust to preferred spice level)
- 4 cups low-sodium chicken broth
- 2 medium potatoes, peeled and diced
- 1 (15-ounce) can corn, drained
- 1/2 cup heavy cream (or full-fat coconut milk)
- Salt, pepper to taste
- Sour cream and chopped chives for garnish

Instructions:

1. Heat olive oil in a large pot. Add onion and celery, saute until softened.
2. Add chicken, paprika, and chili powder. Cook until chicken is browned on all sides.
3. Pour in chicken broth, potatoes, and corn. Bring to a simmer and cook for 15-20 minutes, or until potatoes are tender.
4. Stir in heavy cream and season with salt and pepper.
5. Serve hot, garnished with a dollop of sour cream and chives.

Prep Time: 15 minutes **Cook Time:** 30-35 minutes

Nutritional Info (approx. per serving):

- Calories: 400,
- Sodium: 400mg,
- Potassium: 650mg,
- Fiber: 5g, Protein: 30g

Tips:

- Use leftover cooked chicken or rotisserie chicken for a shortcut.
- Add other POTS-friendly vegetables like chopped bell peppers or carrots.
- Top with crumbled bacon for a flavor boost and extra saltiness.

Hearty Minestrone

- **POTS Power:** This classic is packed with vegetables like carrots, zucchini, and beans, delivering a boost of potassium, fiber, and vitamins. Whole-wheat pasta adds satisfying carbohydrates, and the savory broth provides hydration and sodium.
- **Lunchtime Love:** Minestrone is both comforting and nourishing. Adding a sprinkle of Parmesan cheese on top offers extra saltiness and flavor.

Ingredients:

- 1 tablespoon olive oil
- 1 onion, chopped
- 2 carrots, chopped
- 2 celery stalks, chopped
- 1 zucchini, chopped
- 2 cloves garlic, minced
- 1 (15-ounce) can kidney beans, rinsed and drained
- 1 (15-ounce) can diced tomatoes
- 4 cups vegetable broth
- 1/2 cup small whole-wheat pasta (ditalini, elbows)
- 1/2 teaspoon dried Italian herbs
- Salt, pepper to taste
- Grated Parmesan cheese for garnish

Instructions:

1. Heat olive oil in a large pot. Saute onion, carrots, celery, and zucchini until slightly softened. Add garlic and cook for another minute.
2. Stir in beans, tomatoes, broth, pasta, and Italian herbs. Bring to a simmer and cook for 10-15 minutes, or until pasta is tender and vegetables are cooked through.
3. Season with salt and pepper to taste. Serve hot, garnished with Parmesan cheese.

Prep Time: 10 minutes **Cook Time:** 20-25 minutes

Nutritional Info (approx. per serving):

- Calories: 280,
- Sodium: 400mg,
- Potassium: 650mg,
- Fiber: 10g,
- Protein: 12g

Tips:

- Add other POTS-friendly veggies like chopped spinach, green beans, or bell peppers.
- Use a pre-made low-sodium minestrone soup base for a quick shortcut.
- Top with a dollop of pesto for a burst of fresh flavor.

Chilled Cucumber & Avocado Soup

- **POTS Power:** Cucumber and avocado offer hydration, healthy fats, and a dose of potassium. Yogurt adds creaminess, while lemon and dill provide bright, refreshing flavors.
- **Lunchtime Love:** This chilled soup is perfect for hot days or when you want a lighter, refreshing meal. Serve it with whole-grain crackers or a side salad.

Ingredients:

- 1 large cucumber, peeled, seeded, and chopped
- 1 avocado, chopped
- 1/2 cup plain Greek yogurt
- 1/4 cup fresh dill, chopped
- 2 tablespoons lemon juice
- 1 cup vegetable broth
- Salt, pepper to taste

Instructions:

1. Combine all ingredients in a blender and blend until completely smooth.
2. Chill in the refrigerator for at least 2 hours for flavors to meld.
3. Season with salt and pepper to taste before serving.

Prep Time: 10 minutes **Chill Time:** 2 hours minimum

Nutritional Info (approx. per serving):

- Calories: 200,
- Sodium: 250mg,
- Potassium: 500mg,
- Fiber: 6g,
- Protein: 8g

Tips:

- Garnish with additional dill sprigs or a drizzle of olive oil.
- Add a pinch of cayenne pepper for a subtle kick.
- For extra creaminess, use a dollop of sour cream instead of yogurt.

Salads

Mediterranean Quinoa Salad

- **POTS Power:** Cooked quinoa provides protein and fiber. Cucumber, tomatoes, and olives offer potassium and hydration. Feta cheese boosts saltiness, and the lemon-oregano vinaigrette adds bright flavor.
- **Lunchtime Love:** This salad is light, refreshing, and packed with Mediterranean flavors. Pair with a side of hummus for extra protein and a creamy element.

Ingredients:

- 1 cup cooked quinoa
- 1 cucumber, chopped
- 1 cup cherry tomatoes, halved
- 1/2 cup Kalamata olives, pitted and chopped
- 1/4 cup crumbled feta cheese
- Lemon-Oregano Vinaigrette (recipe below)

Lemon-Oregano Vinaigrette

- 3 tablespoons olive oil
- 2 tablespoons lemon juice
- 1 teaspoon dried oregano
- Pinch of salt, pepper

Instructions:

1. Combine Salad: In a large bowl, combine quinoa, cucumber, tomatoes, olives, and feta cheese.

2. **Make Vinaigrette:** Whisk together olive oil, lemon juice, oregano, salt, and pepper.
3. **Toss to Combine:** Pour vinaigrette over salad and toss to coat evenly. Serve chilled or at room temperature.

Prep Time: 10 minutes

Nutritional Info (approx. per serving):
- Calories: 350,
- Sodium: 400mg,
- Potassium: 500mg,
- Fiber: 8g,
- Protein: 12g

Tips:
- Add other POTS-friendly chopped veggies like bell peppers or artichoke hearts.
- Use a different type of cheese like goat cheese or mozzarella.
- For extra protein, top with grilled chicken or shrimp.

Southwest Black Bean & Avocado Salad

- **POTS Power**: Black beans and corn add fiber and protein. Avocado provides healthy fats and potassium. Bell peppers and the lime-cilantro dressing deliver flavor **and additional nutrients.**
- **Lunchtime Love:** This vibrant salad offers satisfying textures and a burst of Southwest flavors. Top with shredded chicken for extra protein or tortilla chips for a salty crunch.

Ingredients:

- 1 (15-ounce) can black beans, rinsed and drained
- 1 cup corn kernels (fresh or frozen)
- 1 avocado, diced
- 1 bell pepper (any color), diced
- 1/4 cup chopped cilantro
- Lime-Cilantro Dressing (recipe below)

Lime-Cilantro Dressing:

- 3 tablespoons olive oil
- 2 tablespoons lime juice
- 1/4 cup chopped cilantro
- Pinch of salt, pepper, cumin

Instructions

1. Combine Salad: In a bowl, combine black beans, corn, avocado, bell pepper, and cilantro.

2. **Make Dressing:** Whisk together olive oil, lime juice, cilantro, salt, pepper, and cumin.
3. **Assemble:** Toss the salad with the dressing and serve immediately.

Prep Time: 10 minutes

Nutritional Info (approx. per serving): Calories: 320, Sodium: 250mg, Potassium: 700mg, Fiber: 12g, Protein: 10g

Tips:
- Add a sprinkle of chili powder or a dash of hot sauce for spice.
- Top with crumbled queso fresco or cotija cheese for extra saltiness.

Broccoli & Barley Salad

- **POTS Power:** Broccoli is packed with potassium and fiber. Barley provides complex carbohydrates and protein. Almonds offer healthy fats and crunch, cranberries add sweetness, and the tangy dijon vinaigrette delivers bold flavor
- **Lunchtime Love:** This satisfying salad offers a mix of textures and flavors and can be easily customized with your favorite add-ins.

Ingredients:

- 1 cup cooked barley
- 2 cups steamed broccoli florets
- 1/4 cup chopped almonds
- 1/4 cup dried cranberries
- Dijon Vinaigrette (recipe below)

Dijon Vinaigrette:

- 3 tablespoons olive oil
- 2 tablespoons Dijon mustard
- 1 tablespoon lemon juice
- Pinch of salt, pepper

Instructions:

1. **Combine Salad:** In a large bowl, combine cooked barley, broccoli, almonds, and cranberries.
2. **Make Vinaigrette:** Whisk together olive oil, Dijon mustard, lemon juice, salt, and pepper.
3. **Toss & Serve:** Pour vinaigrette over salad and toss to coat. Serve chilled or at room temperature.

Prep Time: 10 minutes (plus barley cooking time)

Nutritional Info (approx. per serving):

- Calories: 380,
- Sodium: 200mg,
- Potassium: 550mg,
- Fiber: 9g,
- Protein: 10g

Tips:

- Add other POTS-friendly vegetables like chopped cucumbers, bell peppers, or shredded carrots.
- Use another type of grain like quinoa or farro in place of barley.
- Top with crumbled feta or goat cheese for extra saltiness.

Asian Noodle Salad

- **POTS Power:** Rice noodles offer carbohydrates, edamame adds protein, and the vegetables contribute potassium and fiber. The sesame-ginger dressing provides a boost of flavor.
- **Lunchtime Love:** This light and refreshing salad is packed with Asian-inspired flavors. Add grilled chicken, tofu, or shrimp for an extra protein boost.

Ingredients:

- 8 ounces rice noodles
- 1 cup shredded cabbage
- 1 cup shredded carrots
- 1 cup shelled edamame (frozen or fresh)
- Sesame-Ginger Dressing (recipe below)

Sesame-Ginger Dressing:

- 3 tablespoons soy sauce (reduced-sodium)
- 2 tablespoons rice vinegar
- 1 tablespoon sesame oil
- 1 teaspoon grated fresh ginger
- Pinch of red pepper flakes (optional)

Instructions:

1. **Cook & Combine:** Cook rice noodles according to package directions. Combine with cabbage, carrots, and edamame in a bowl.
2. **Make Dressing:** Whisk together all dressing ingredients.

3. **Assemble:** Toss salad with dressing. Serve chilled or at room temperature.

Prep Time: 15 minutes

Nutritional Info (approx. per serving):

- Calories: 300,
- Sodium: 400mg,
- Potassium: 450mg,
- Fiber: 8g,
- Protein: 12g

Tips:

- Add other POTS-friendly chopped veggies like cucumbers, bell peppers, or snap peas.
- Use a different type of noodle like soba or udon.
- Top with chopped peanuts or cashews for extra crunch

Kale & Lentil Salad

- **POTS Power:** Kale delivers potassium, fiber, and antioxidants. Lentils provide protein and iron. Feta contributes saltiness, cranberries add sweetness, and walnuts offer healthy fats for a balanced meal.
- **Lunchtime Love:** This hearty salad keeps you feeling full and energized. The lemon vinaigrette adds bright, zesty flavor.

Ingredients:

- 1 bunch kale, stems removed, leaves chopped
- 1 cup cooked lentils
- 1/4 cup crumbled feta cheese
- 1/4 cup dried cranberries
- 1/4 cup chopped walnuts
- Lemon Vinaigrette (recipe below)

Lemon Vinaigrette:

- 3 tablespoons olive oil
- 2 tablespoons lemon juice
- 1 teaspoon honey (or maple syrup)
- Pinch of salt, pepper

Instructions:

1. **Massage the Kale:** Place chopped kale in a bowl. Drizzle with a bit of olive oil and lemon juice. Massage with your hands for 1-2 minutes to soften the leaves.

2. **Combine Salad:** Add cooked lentils, feta, cranberries, and walnuts to the kale.
3. **Make Vinaigrette:** Whisk together olive oil, lemon juice, honey, salt, and pepper.
4. **Assemble:** Toss the salad with the vinaigrette. Serve chilled or at room temperature.

Prep Time: 15 minutes

Nutritional Info (approx. per serving):
- Calories: 350,
- Sodium: 350mg,
- Potassium: 700mg,
- Fiber: 9g,
- Protein: 15g

Tips:
- Use another type of hearty green like spinach or Swiss chard instead of kale.
- Substitute feta with another salty cheese like goat cheese or Parmesan.
- Add other POTS-friendly chopped vegetables like cucumbers, bell peppers, or cherry tomatoes.

Main Dishes

Tuna Salad Lettuce Wraps

- **POTS Power:** Tuna is a good source of protein and offers some natural sodium. Pairing it with Dijon mustard and celery adds flavor and crunch. Lettuce wraps provide a lighter alternative to bread.
- **Lunchtime Love:** This classic lunch is quick, easy, and customizable. Perfect for those days when you want something satisfying without the heaviness of bread.

Ingredients:

- 1 (5-ounce) can tuna, drained
- 2 tablespoons mayonnaise
- 1 tablespoon Dijon mustard
- 1 celery stalk, finely chopped
- Salt, pepper to taste
- Large lettuce leaves (butter lettuce, romaine, etc.)

Instructions:

1. Mix Tuna Salad: In a bowl, combine tuna, mayonnaise, Dijon mustard, celery, salt, and pepper. Mash slightly for a chunkier texture or mix well for a smoother salad.
2. Assemble: Spoon tuna salad onto lettuce leaves. Wrap and enjoy!

Prep Time: 10 minutes

Nutritional Info (approx. per 2 lettuce wraps):

- Calories: 250, Sodium: 350mg, Potassium: 300mg, Fiber: 2g, Protein: 20g

Tips:

- Add other chopped veggies like cucumbers, bell peppers, or olives.
- Use avocado mayonnaise for extra creaminess and healthy fats.
- Serve with a side of whole-grain crackers for those who want some extra carbs.

Chicken & Veggie Stuffed Peppers

- **POTS Power:** Ground chicken provides protein, peppers offer potassium and vitamins, quinoa boosts fiber and protein, and marinara adds flavor. The sprinkle of mozzarella provides a salty kick.
- **Lunchtime Love:** These stuffed peppers are both comforting and nutritious. Bake a batch ahead of time for easy, re-heatable lunches.

Ingredients:

- 4 bell peppers (any color), halved lengthwise and seeded
- 1 pound ground chicken
- 1/2 cup cooked quinoa
- 1/2 cup chopped spinach
- 1 jar marinara sauce
- 1/2 cup shredded mozzarella cheese
- Salt, pepper, Italian herbs to taste

Instructions:

1. Preheat & Prep: Preheat oven to 400°F (200°C). Lightly oil a baking dish.
2. Cook Filling: Brown ground chicken in a skillet. Stir in quinoa, spinach, ½ cup marinara, and season with salt, pepper, and herbs.

3. **Stuff Peppers:** Fill pepper halves with chicken mixture. Place in oiled baking dish and top with remaining marinara sauce.
4. **Bake & Cheese:** Bake for 25-30 minutes, then sprinkle with mozzarella. Bake for an additional 5 minutes until cheese is melted.

Prep Time: 15 minutes Cook Time: 30-35 minutes

Nutritional Info (approx. per stuffed pepper half):

- Calories: 350, Sodium: 450mg, Potassium: 600mg, Fiber: 8g, Protein: 30g

Tips:

- Substitute ground turkey or another lean protein for the chicken.
- Add other POTS-friendly veggies like diced zucchini or mushrooms.
- Use a low-sodium marinara sauce.

Quinoa Veggie Burgers

- **POTS Power**: Quinoa and black beans provide protein and fiber, while vegetables offer potassium and other nutrients. Spices add flavor, and avocado spread boosts healthy fats.
- **Lunchtime Love**: These hearty veggie burgers are a delicious and satisfying alternative to traditional beef burgers. Serve them on whole-wheat buns for a complete meal.

Ingredients (for the patties):

- 1 cup cooked quinoa
- 1 (15-ounce) can black beans, rinsed and drained
- 1/2 cup chopped onion
- 1/2 cup chopped bell pepper
- 1 egg
- 1/4 cup breadcrumbs
- 1 teaspoon chili powder
- 1/2 teaspoon cumin
- Salt, pepper to taste

Toppings:

- Whole-wheat buns
- Avocado spread (mashed avocado with salt, pepper, and a squeeze of lime juice)
- Lettuce
- Tomato slices

Instructions:

1. **Mash & Mix:** In a bowl, mash black beans slightly. Add quinoa, onion, bell pepper, egg, breadcrumbs, spices, salt, and pepper. Mix until well combined.
2. **Form Patties:** Shape mixture into 4-6 patties.
3. **Cook:** Heat a skillet with oil. Cook patties for 4-5 minutes per side, or until golden brown and heated through.
4. **Assemble:** Serve patties on buns with avocado spread, lettuce, tomato, and your favorite toppings.

Prep Time: 15 minutes Cook Time: 15 minutes

Nutritional Info (approx. per burger):

- Calories: 300, Sodium: 300mg, Potassium: 550mg, Fiber: 10g, Protein: 15g

Tips:

- Add other POTS-friendly chopped veggies like carrots, zucchini, or mushrooms.
- Use gluten-free breadcrumbs if needed.
- Top with a dollop of Greek yogurt or a sprinkle of crumbled feta for extra saltiness.

Shrimp Scampi with Zucchini Noodles

- **POTS Power:** Shrimp offers protein, zucchini provides potassium and fiber, while the garlic, lemon, and white wine sauce delivers flavor.
- **Lunchtime** Love: This light and flavorful dish is perfect for a warm-weather lunch or when you want a lighter take on pasta.

Ingredients

- 1 pound shrimp, peeled and deveined
- 2 medium zucchini, spiralized
- 2 tablespoons olive oil
- 3 cloves garlic, minced
- 1/4 cup dry white wine
- 1/4 cup lemon juice
- 1/4 cup chopped fresh parsley
- Salt, pepper to taste

Instructions

1. Prep Zucchini Noodles: Spiralize zucchini or use pre-made zucchini noodles.
2. Sauté Shrimp: Season shrimp with salt and pepper. Heat 1 tablespoon of oil in a skillet and cook shrimp 2-3 minutes per side until pink. Remove and set aside.

3. **Make Sauce:** Add remaining oil to skillet. Sauté garlic briefly. Deglaze pan with white wine and lemon juice, scraping browned bits. Let simmer 1-2 minutes.
4. **Combine:** Add zucchini noodles and shrimp. Toss to coat, cooking noodles until just tender. Stir in parsley, season with salt and pepper.

Prep Time: 10 minutes Cook Time: 10 minutes

Nutritional Info (approx. per serving):
- Calories: 250,
- Sodium: 400mg,
- Potassium: 600mg,
- Fiber: 5g,
- Protein: 25g

Tips:
- Substitute with another protein like scallops or chicken.
- Add a pinch of red pepper flakes for a bit of heat.
- Serve with a sprinkle of Parmesan cheese for extra saltiness.

Salmon & Roasted Veggie Bowls

- **POTS Power:** Salmon provides protein and healthy fats, while sweet potatoes and Brussels sprouts deliver potassium, fiber, and vitamins. The balsamic glaze adds a touch of sweetness and tanginess.
- **Lunchtime Love:** This dish is satisfying, packed with nutrients, and easy to customize with your favorite vegetables. The vibrant colors make it a feast for the eyes too!

Ingredients:

- 1 pound salmon fillet, cut into portions
- 1 pound sweet potatoes, peeled and diced
- 1 pound Brussels sprouts, trimmed and halved
- 2 tablespoons olive oil
- Salt, pepper, your favorite herbs (thyme, rosemary) to taste
- 1/4 cup balsamic vinegar

Instructions:

1. Preheat & Prep: Preheat oven to 425°F (220°C). Toss sweet potatoes and Brussels sprouts with 1 tablespoon of olive oil, salt, pepper, and herbs on a baking sheet.
2. Roast Veggies: Roast vegetables for 20 minutes.
3. Cook Salmon: While veggies roast, season salmon with salt and pepper. Heat remaining olive oil in a skillet and cook

salmon, skin-side down first, for 3-4 minutes per side, or until cooked through.

4. **Make Glaze:** Towards the end of the cooking time, add balsamic vinegar to the skillet with the salmon and let it reduce slightly to create a glaze.
5. **Assemble Bowls:** Divide roasted vegetables among bowls. Top with salmon and drizzle with the balsamic glaze.

Prep Time: 15 minutes Cook Time: 25-30 minutes

Nutritional Info (approx. per serving):

- Calories: 450, Sodium: 350mg, Potassium: 800mg, Fiber: 10g, Protein: 35g

Tips:

- Substitute with another type of fish, like cod or halibut.
- Use other POTS-friendly vegetables like broccoli, carrots, or bell peppers.
- Top with a sprinkle of feta cheese or chopped nuts for extra flavor and saltiness.

Chapter 4: Easy and Nourishing Dinners

Flavor-Packed Mains

One-Pan Roasted Chicken & Veggies

- **POTS Power:** Chicken provides protein, while sweet potatoes and Brussels sprouts offer potassium, fiber, and vitamins. Simple herbs and spices add flavor without excessive sodium.
- **Dinner Delight:** This dish is easy, satisfying, and packed with flavor. It's a one-pan wonder, perfect for busy weeknights.

Ingredients:

- 4 bone-in, skin-on chicken thighs
- 1 pound sweet potatoes, peeled and diced
- 1 pound Brussels sprouts, trimmed and halved
- 1 onion, sliced
- 2 tablespoons olive oil
- Salt, pepper, your favorite herbs (like thyme, rosemary, or a poultry seasoning blend)

Instructions
1. Preheat oven to 425°F (220°C).
2. In a large bowl, toss chicken, sweet potatoes, Brussels sprouts, and onion with olive oil, salt, pepper, and herbs.
3. Spread the mixture evenly onto a baking sheet.
4. Roast for 30-35 minutes, or until chicken is cooked through and vegetables are tender and slightly browned.
5. Serve immediately with a side of quinoa or your favorite grain for added protein and fiber.

Prep Time: 15 minutes **Cook Time:** 30-35 minutes

Nutritional Info (approx. per serving):
- Calories: 400, Sodium: 350mg, Potassium: 750mg, Fiber: 8g, Protein: 30g

Tips:
- Use boneless, skinless chicken thighs or breasts for a quicker cook time.
- Add other POTS-friendly vegetables like carrots, parsnips, or bell peppers.
- For a flavor boost, toss veggies with a drizzle of balsamic vinegar in addition to the herbs.

Sheet-Pan Salmon with Lemon & Asparagus

- **POTS Power:** Salmon is rich in protein and healthy fats, asparagus offers potassium and fiber, while lemon and dill provide bright, fresh flavors.
- **Dinner Delight:** This quick and easy dish is perfect for weeknights. Customize it with your favorite seasonings.

Ingredients:

- 1 pound salmon fillet, cut into portions
- 1 pound asparagus, trimmed
- 2 tablespoons olive oil
- 1 lemon, sliced
- 2 tablespoons fresh dill (or 1 teaspoon dried dill)
- Salt, pepper to taste

Instructions:

1. Preheat oven to 400°F (200°C).
2. Toss asparagus with 1 tablespoon of olive oil, salt, and pepper, and arrange on a baking sheet.
3. Season salmon with salt, pepper, and dill. Place on the baking sheet alongside asparagus. Top with lemon slices.
4. Bake for 12-15 minutes, or until salmon is cooked through and asparagus is tender-crisp.

Prep Time: 10 minutes **Cook Time:** 12-15 minutes

Nutritional Info (approx. per serving):

- Calories: 350, Sodium: 250mg, Potassium: 600mg, Fiber: 5g, Protein: 35g

Tips

- Substitute with another firm white fish, like cod or halibut.
- Add baby potatoes to the pan for extra heartiness.
- Swap dill for other herbs like rosemary or thyme.

Lentil & Mushroom "Shepherd's Pie"

- **POTS Power:** Lentils provide protein and fiber, while mushrooms add earthy flavor and potassium. Mashed sweet potatoes offer a boost of vitamins and a touch of sweetness.
- **Dinner Delight:** A comforting and hearty vegetarian take on the classic Shepherd's Pie – perfect for chilly evenings.

Ingredients:

- 1 tablespoon olive oil
- 1 onion, chopped
- 2 cloves garlic, minced
- 1 pound mushrooms, chopped
- 1 cup dried lentils
- 3 cups vegetable broth
- 1 teaspoon dried thyme
- Salt, pepper to taste
- Mashed Sweet Potato Topping (recipe below)

Mashed Sweet Potato Topping:

- 2 large sweet potatoes, peeled and diced
- 1/4 cup milk (or unsweetened plant-based milk)
- 2 tablespoons butter (or olive oil)
- Salt, pepper to taste

Instructions:

1. **Cook Lentils:** Saute onion and garlic in olive oil until softened. Add mushrooms and cook until browned. Stir in lentils, broth, thyme, salt, and pepper. Bring to a simmer, then reduce heat and simmer for 25-30 minutes, or until lentils are tender.
2. **Make Topping:** While lentils cook, boil sweet potatoes until fork-tender. Drain, then mash with milk, butter (or olive oil), salt, and pepper.
3. **Assemble:** Preheat oven to 400°F (200°C). Pour lentil mixture into a baking dish. Spread mashed sweet potatoes over the top.
4. **Bake:** Bake for 15-20 minutes, or until topping is heated through and lightly browned.

Prep Time: 20 minutes **Cook Time:** 40-45 minutes

Nutritional Info (approx. per serving):

- Calories: 400, Sodium: 300mg, Potassium: 900mg, Fiber: 15g, Protein: 20g

Tips:

- Add other chopped vegetables like carrots, celery, or zucchini.
- Use a low-sodium vegetable broth.
- Top with a sprinkle of Parmesan cheese for extra saltiness and flavor.

Spicy Shrimp & Quinoa Stir-Fry

- **POTS Power:** Shrimp is a good source of protein, bell peppers and broccoli offer potassium and vitamins, while quinoa provides fiber and additional protein. The spicy sauce adds flavor and a touch of warmth.
- **Dinner Delight:** This quick and flavorful stir-fry is perfect for weeknights and easily customizable with your favorite vegetables.

Ingredients:

- 1 pound shrimp, peeled and deveined
- 1 tablespoon olive oil
- 1 bell pepper (any color), sliced
- 1 cup broccoli florets
- 1/2 cup cooked quinoa
- Spicy Stir-Fry Sauce (recipe below)

Spicy Stir-Fry Sauce

- 2 tablespoons soy sauce (reduced-sodium)
- 2 tablespoons rice vinegar
- 1 tablespoon sesame oil
- 1 teaspoon honey (or maple syrup)
- 1 teaspoon grated fresh ginger
- 1/2 teaspoon red pepper flakes (adjust to taste)

Instructions
1. **Make Sauce:** Whisk together all sauce ingredients.
2. **Stir-Fry:** Heat olive oil in a large skillet. Add shrimp and cook until pink. Remove and set aside.
3. Add bell pepper and broccoli to the skillet. Cook until tender-crisp.
4. Return shrimp to the pan along with cooked quinoa. Pour in the sauce and toss to coat. Cook for 1-2 minutes until heated through.

Prep Time: 10 minutes **Cook Time:** 15 minutes

Nutritional Info (approx. per serving):
- Calories: 350, Sodium: 450mg, Potassium: 550mg, Fiber: 8g, Protein: 30g

Tips:
- Substitute with chicken, tofu, or another protein of choice.
- Add other POTS-friendly vegetables like snap peas, carrots, or edamame.
- Adjust the spice level to your liking.

Turkey Meatballs with Zucchini Noodles

- **POTS Power:** Lean turkey provides protein, zucchini noodles offer a lighter alternative to pasta, and Italian herbs and marinara add flavor.
- **Dinner Delight:** This dish offers classic flavors while sneaking in extra veggies. Perfect for weeknights or when you crave something comforting yet balanced.

Ingredients:

Meatballs:

- 1 pound lean ground turkey
- 1/2 cup breadcrumbs
- 1/4 cup grated Parmesan cheese
- 1 egg
- 1 tablespoon dried Italian herbs
- Salt, pepper to taste

Other:

- 2 tablespoons olive oil
- 1 jar marinara sauce
- 4 medium zucchini, spiralized

Instructions:

1. **Make Meatballs:** Combine turkey, breadcrumbs, Parmesan, egg, herbs, salt, and pepper in a bowl. Mix gently and form into meatballs (about 1-inch each).

2. **Cook Meatballs:** Heat olive oil in a large skillet. Brown meatballs on all sides. Add marinara sauce and simmer for 15-20 minutes, or until meatballs are cooked through.
3. **Prepare Zucchini Noodles:** While meatballs cook, lightly saute the zucchini noodles in a separate pan with a bit of olive oil, just until tender-crisp.
4. **Assemble:** Divide zucchini noodles among bowls. Top with meatballs and sauce. Sprinkle with additional Parmesan cheese if desired.

Prep Time: 15 minutes **Cook Time:** 25-30 minutes

Nutritional Info (approx. per serving):

- Calories: 400, Sodium: 500mg, Potassium: 650mg, Fiber: 8g, Protein: 35g

Tips:

- Use a low-sodium marinara sauce.
- Add other chopped vegetables to the marinara sauce, like onions, bell peppers, or mushrooms.
- Serve with a side of whole-wheat garlic bread for dipping into the sauce.

Light & Refreshing

Mediterranean Chickpea Salad Pitas

- **POTS Power:** Chickpeas offer protein and fiber, cucumbers and tomatoes provide hydration and potassium, olives add healthy fats, and feta delivers saltiness. The lemon vinaigrette adds bright, zesty flavor.
- **Dinner Delight:** This vibrant and flavorful salad is perfect for a light yet satisfying meal. Serve with whole-wheat pitas for a complete and balanced dinner.

Ingredients:

- 1 (15-ounce) can chickpeas, rinsed and drained
- 1 cup chopped cucumber
- 1 cup halved cherry tomatoes
- 1/2 cup crumbled feta cheese
- 1/4 cup Kalamata olives, pitted and chopped
- Lemon Vinaigrette (recipe below)
- Whole-wheat pitas

Lemon Vinaigrette:

- 3 tablespoons olive oil
- 2 tablespoons lemon juice
- 1 teaspoon dried oregano
- Salt, pepper to taste

Instructions:

1. **Make Salad:** Combine chickpeas, cucumber, tomatoes, feta, and olives in a bowl.
2. **Make Vinaigrette:** Whisk together olive oil, lemon juice, oregano, salt, and pepper.
3. **Assemble:** Toss salad with vinaigrette. Serve inside warmed whole-wheat pitas.

Prep Time: 10 minutes

Nutritional Info (approx. per serving with 1 pita):

- Calories: 400, Sodium: 550mg, Potassium: 600mg, Fiber: 10g, Protein: 18g

Tips:

- Add other POTS-friendly chopped veggies like bell peppers or artichoke hearts.
- Use a different type of cheese like goat cheese or mozzarella.
- Top with a dollop of hummus for extra protein and creaminess.

Summer Veggie Frittata

- **POTS Power:** Eggs provide protein, while zucchini, squash, and bell peppers offer potassium, vitamins, and fiber. Parmesan adds a touch of saltiness and richness.
- **Dinner Delight:** This fluffy frittata is versatile and easy to customize. Perfect for a light dinner, a satisfying brunch, or even cut into squares for a healthy snack.

Ingredients:

- 1 tablespoon olive oil
- 1/2 cup chopped onion
- 1/2 cup chopped zucchini
- 1/2 cup chopped yellow squash
- 1/2 cup chopped bell pepper (any color)
- 8 eggs
- 1/4 cup milk (or unsweetened plant-based milk)
- 1/4 cup grated Parmesan cheese
- Salt, pepper to taste

Instructions:

1. **Sauté Veggies:** Heat olive oil in an oven-safe skillet. Saute onion until softened, then add zucchini, squash, and bell pepper. Cook until tender-crisp.
2. **Whisk Eggs:** In a bowl, whisk together eggs, milk, Parmesan cheese, salt, and pepper.

3. **Pour & Bake:** Pour egg mixture over vegetables in the skillet. Cook over medium-low heat for few minutes, until edges start to set.
4. **Finish in Oven:** Transfer skillet to preheated 350°F (180°C) oven. Bake for 10-15 minutes, or until frittata is set and puffed.

Prep Time: 15 minutes **Cook Time:** 20-25 minutes

Nutritional Info (approx. per serving):

- Calories: 200, Sodium: 300mg, Potassium: 450mg, Fiber: 4g, Protein: 15g

Tips:

- Add other POTS-friendly vegetables like spinach, mushrooms, or tomatoes.
- Use a reduced-sodium milk.
- Top with a sprinkle of feta cheese or a dollop of Greek yogurt for extra flavor and saltiness.

Asian-Inspired Lettuce Wraps

- **POTS Power:** Ground chicken or tofu provides protein, carrots and rice noodles offer complex carbs, and the lettuce cups are a refreshing and hydrating base. The peanut sauce adds healthy fats and a delicious savory-sweet flavor.
- **Dinner Delight:** These customizable wraps are fun to assemble and deliver great flavor combinations.

Ingredients:

- 1 tablespoon olive oil
- 1 pound ground chicken (or crumbled tofu)
- 1 clove garlic, minced
- 1 tablespoon grated fresh ginger
- 2 tablespoons soy sauce (reduced-sodium)
- 1 bag coleslaw mix (or shredded carrots and cabbage)
- 1/2 cup cooked rice noodles
- Large lettuce leaves (butter lettuce, bibb, or romaine)
- Chopped peanuts, scallions, cilantro for garnish
- Peanut Sauce (recipe below)

Peanut Sauce:

- 1/4 cup creamy peanut butter
- 2 tablespoons soy sauce (reduced-sodium)
- 1 tablespoon rice vinegar
- 1 tablespoon honey (or maple syrup)
- 1 teaspoon grated fresh ginger

- Hot sauce or chili flakes to taste (optional)

Instructions:

1. **Cook Protein:** Heat olive oil in a skillet. Cook ground chicken (or tofu), garlic, and ginger until cooked through. Stir in soy sauce.
2. **Make Peanut Sauce:** Whisk together all sauce ingredients, adding a splash of water to thin if needed.
3. **Combine Filling:** In a bowl, combine cooked protein with coleslaw mix and rice noodles.
4. **Assemble:** Spoon filling into lettuce leaves. Garnish with peanuts, scallions, cilantro, and drizzle with peanut sauce.

Prep Time: 15 minutes **Cook Time:** 15 minutes

Nutritional Info (approx. per 2 lettuce wraps):

- Calories: 350, Sodium: 500mg, Potassium: 400mg, Fiber: 6g, Protein: 25g

Tips:

- Substitute with another lean protein like shrimp or ground turkey.
- Add other chopped POTS-friendly vegetables to the filling, like bell peppers or snap peas.
- Adjust the spiciness of the peanut sauce to your liking.

Avocado & Black Bean Quesadillas

- **POTS Power:** Black beans provide protein and fiber, avocado offers healthy fats, corn adds sweetness, and cheese delivers saltiness. Whole-wheat tortillas boost fiber intake.
- **Dinner Delight:** These quesadillas are quick, easy, and so satisfying. Perfect for a weeknight meal or a fun, customizable snack.

Ingredients:

- 1 tablespoon olive oil
- 1/2 onion, chopped
- 1 (15-ounce) can black beans, rinsed and drained
- 1 cup corn kernels (fresh or frozen)
- 1/2 teaspoon chili powder
- 1/2 teaspoon cumin
- 4 (8-inch) whole-wheat tortillas
- 1 cup shredded cheese (cheddar, Monterey Jack, or a blend)
- 1 avocado, mashed
- Salsa and sour cream for serving (optional)

Instructions:

1. **Cook Filling:** Heat olive oil in a skillet. Sauté onion until softened. Add black beans, corn, chili powder, and cumin. Cook for a few minutes to warm through.
2. **Assemble:** Spread half of each tortilla with mashed avocado. Top with bean mixture and cheese. Fold tortillas in half.

3. **Cook Quesadillas:** Heat a dry skillet. Cook quesadillas one or two at a time, for 1-2 minutes per side until golden and cheese is melted.
4. **Serve:** Cut into wedges and serve with salsa and sour cream (if desired).

Prep Time: 10 minutes **Cook Time:** 15 minutes

Nutritional Info (approx. per 2 wedges):

- Calories: 450, Sodium: 450mg, Potassium: 650mg, Fiber: 12g, Protein: 20g

Tips:

- Add other POTS-friendly chopped vegetables to the filling, like bell peppers, spinach, or zucchini.
- Use a low-sodium canned black bean option.
- Top with a sprinkle of crumbled feta or cotija cheese for extra saltiness.

Tuna Nicoise Salad

- **POTS Power:** Tuna is a good source of protein and offers natural sodium. Potatoes, green beans, olives, and hard-boiled eggs provide nutrients, while the tangy vinaigrette balances flavors.
- **Dinner Delight:** This composed salad is elegant yet surprisingly easy to assemble. It's a complete meal packed with flavor and textures.

Ingredients:

- 4 small red potatoes, boiled and quartered
- 1/2 pound green beans, trimmed and blanched
- 2 hard-boiled eggs, quartered
- 1 (5-ounce) can tuna, drained
- 1/2 cup Kalamata olives, pitted
- 4 cups mixed greens
- Vinaigrette (recipe below)

Vinaigrette:

- 3 tablespoons olive oil
- 2 tablespoons red wine vinegar
- 1 teaspoon Dijon mustard
- Salt, pepper to taste

Instructions:

1. **Prep Veggies:** Boil potatoes until tender, then quarter them. Blanch green beans briefly in boiling water, then cool in ice water to stop cooking.
2. **Hard-Boil Eggs:** Cook eggs to desired doneness, peel, and quarter.
3. **Make Vinaigrette:** Whisk together olive oil, red wine vinegar, Dijon mustard, salt, and pepper.
4. **Assemble:** Arrange greens on a platter. Top with potatoes, green beans, hard-boiled eggs, tuna, and olives. Drizzle with vinaigrette just before serving.

Prep Time: 15 minutes **Cook Time:** 15-20 minutes (for potatoes and eggs)

Nutritional Info (approx. per serving):

- Calories: 350, Sodium: 450mg, Potassium: 700mg, Fiber: 8g, Protein: 25g

Tips:

- Use other firm, white fish instead of tuna if you prefer.
- Add other POTS-friendly vegetables like cherry tomatoes, cucumbers, or radishes.
- Top with a sprinkle of capers for an extra briny kick.

Hearty & Comforting

Chicken Pot Pie with Sweet Potato Crust

- **POTS Power:** Chicken provides protein, the savory filling offers vegetables like carrots and peas, while the sweet potato crust delivers potassium and a touch of sweetness.
- **Dinner Delight:** This twist on the classic comfort food is both satisfying and nourishing. The sweet potato crust adds a unique flavor and extra nutrients.

Ingredients:

Filling:

- 1 tablespoon olive oil
- 1 onion, chopped
- 2 carrots, chopped
- 2 stalks celery, chopped
- 2 cloves garlic, minced
- 2 cups cooked chicken, shredded
- 1/2 cup frozen peas
- 1/4 cup all-purpose flour
- 2 cups low-sodium chicken broth
- 1/2 cup milk (or unsweetened plant-based milk)
- Salt, pepper, and herbs (like thyme or parsley) to taste

Sweet Potato Crust:

- 2 large sweet potatoes, peeled and diced
- 1/4 cup milk (or unsweetened plant-based milk)

- 2 tablespoons butter (or olive oil)
- Salt, pepper to taste

Instructions:

1. **Make Filling:** Heat olive oil in a large pot. Saute onion, carrots, celery, and garlic until softened. Add shredded chicken, peas, and flour. Cook for a minute, then stir in chicken broth and milk. Simmer until thickened, then season with salt, pepper, and herbs.
2. **Make Crust:** Boil sweet potatoes, then mash with milk, butter (or olive oil), salt, and pepper.
3. **Assemble:** Preheat oven to 400°F (200°C). Pour filling into a baking dish. Spread mashed sweet potato over the top.
4. **Bake:** Bake for 20-25 minutes, or until topping is golden and heated through.

Prep Time: 20 minutes **Cook Time:** 40-45 minutes

Nutritional Info (approx. per serving):

- Calories: 450, Sodium: 400mg, Potassium: 800mg, Fiber: 8g, Protein: 30g

Tips:

- Add other POTS-friendly chopped vegetables to the filling, like mushrooms or corn.
- Use store-bought rotisserie chicken for a shortcut.
- Brush the sweet potato topping with a beaten egg before baking for a golden, shiny crust.

Slow Cooker Beef Stew

- **POTS Power:** Beef provides protein and iron, while carrots, potatoes, and the rich broth offer satisfying nutrients and hydration.
- **Dinner Delight:** This classic stew is the ultimate comfort food, made extra easy with the slow cooker. Let it simmer all day for tender, flavorful results.

Ingredients:
- 2 pounds beef stew meat, cut into cubes
- 1 tablespoon olive oil
- 1 onion, chopped
- 3 carrots, chopped
- 3 stalks celery, chopped
- 2 cloves garlic, minced
- 4 cups low-sodium beef broth
- 2 medium potatoes, peeled and cubed
- 1 teaspoon dried thyme
- Salt, pepper to taste

Instructions:
1. **Brown Beef:** Season beef with salt and pepper. Brown in olive oil in a skillet. Transfer to slow cooker.
2. **Add Veggies:** Add onion, carrots, celery, and garlic to the slow cooker. Pour in beef broth, potatoes, and thyme. Season with salt and pepper.

3. **Slow Cook:** Cook on LOW for 6-8 hours, or on HIGH for 3-4 hours, until beef is tender.

Prep Time: 15 minutes **Cook Time:** 6-8 hours on LOW or 3-4 hours on HIGH

Nutritional Info (approx. per serving):
- Calories: 400, Sodium: 350mg, Potassium: 700mg, Fiber: 6g, Protein: 35g

Tips:
- Use a low-sodium beef broth.
- Add other POTS-friendly vegetables like parsnips, turnips, or mushrooms.
- Thicken the stew with a slurry of flour and water at the end of cooking if desired.

Vegetarian Chili

- **POTS Power:** This chili is packed with beans (kidney and black beans provide a good mix), offering protein and fiber. Corn adds sweetness, tomatoes offer potassium and vitamins, and the spices deliver warmth and flavor.
- **Dinner Delight:** A satisfying and flavorful chili that's perfect for chilly nights. The toppings let you customize it to your liking and maximize those POTS-friendly additions!

Ingredients:

- 1 tablespoon olive oil
- 1 onion, chopped
- 2 cloves garlic, minced
- 1 green bell pepper, chopped
- 1 (15-ounce) can kidney beans, rinsed and drained
- 1 (15-ounce) can black beans, rinsed and drained
- 1 (15-ounce) can diced tomatoes
- 1 (15-ounce) can corn, drained
- 2 cups vegetable broth
- 2 tablespoons chili powder
- 1 teaspoon cumin
- Salt, pepper to taste
- Toppings: Chopped avocado, shredded cheese, sour cream, chopped cilantro

Instructions:
1. **Sauté Veggies:** Heat olive oil in a large pot. Saute onion, garlic, and bell pepper until softened.
2. **Combine:** Add kidney beans, black beans, tomatoes, corn, broth, chili powder, cumin, salt, and pepper to the pot. Bring to a simmer and cook for 20-30 minutes, or until flavors meld and chili thickens.
3. **Serve:** Ladle chili into bowls and top with your desired toppings.

Prep Time: 10 minutes **Cook Time:** 30 minutes

Nutritional Info (approx. per serving):
- Calories: 350, Sodium: 350mg, Potassium: 800mg, Fiber: 15g, Protein: 20g

Tips:
- Add other POTS-friendly chopped vegetables like carrots, zucchini, or sweet potatoes.
- Adjust the chili powder level to control the spice.
- Serve with a side of whole-grain cornbread or brown rice for a complete meal.

Lentil & Butternut Squash "Lasagna"

- **POTS Power:** Lentils provide protein and fiber, butternut squash offers potassium and vitamins, and ricotta cheese adds creaminess and a touch of saltiness. Marinara contributes flavor and additional nutrients.
- **Dinner Delight:** This healthy twist on lasagna is just as comforting. Layer it up for a satisfying and nourishing meal.

Ingredients:

- 1 tablespoon olive oil
- 1 onion, chopped
- 2 cloves garlic, minced
- 1 cup dried lentils
- 3 cups vegetable broth
- 1 (15-ounce) can marinara sauce
- 1 medium butternut squash, peeled, seeded, and thinly sliced
- 1 (15-ounce) container ricotta cheese
- 1/2 cup shredded mozzarella cheese

Instructions:

1. **Cook Lentils:** Saute onion and garlic in olive oil. Add lentils and broth. Bring to a simmer, then reduce heat and cook until tender (about 20 minutes). Stir in marinara sauce.
2. **Roast Squash:** While lentils cook, toss butternut squash slices with a drizzle of olive oil, salt, and pepper. Roast at 400°F (200°C) for 15-20 minutes, or until tender.

3. **Assemble:** Preheat oven to 375°F (190°C). In a baking dish, layer lentils, squash, ricotta, repeating layers. Top with mozzarella cheese.
4. **Bake:** Bake for 20-25 minutes, or until heated through and cheese is melted.

Prep Time: 20 minutes **Cook Time:** 40-45 minutes

Nutritional Info (approx. per serving):

- Calories: 400, Sodium: 450mg, Potassium: 900mg, Fiber: 12g, Protein: 22g

Tips:

- Use a low-sodium marinara sauce and vegetable broth.
- Add other POTS-friendly vegetables like chopped spinach or mushrooms to the lentil mixture.
- Top with a sprinkle of Parmesan cheese for extra saltiness.

Stuffed Acorn Squash

- **POTS Power:** Acorn squash is rich in potassium and fiber. Quinoa provides protein and additional fiber, ground turkey delivers protein, and the cranberries and walnuts add sweetness, crunch, and healthy fats.
- **Dinner Delight:** These stuffed squash halves make a beautiful presentation and offer a balance of savory and sweet flavors. It's a comforting and satisfying fall or winter meal.

Ingredients:

- 2 acorn squash, halved and seeded
- 1 tablespoon olive oil
- 1 pound ground turkey
- 1 onion, chopped
- 2 cloves garlic, minced
- 1 cup cooked quinoa
- 1/2 cup dried cranberries
- 1/4 cup chopped walnuts
- 1 teaspoon dried sage (or poultry seasoning blend)
- Salt, pepper to taste
- 1/2 cup crumbled feta cheese (optional)

Instructions:
1. **Roast Squash:** Preheat oven to 400°F (200°C). Drizzle cut sides of squash with olive oil, season with salt and pepper. Place cut-side down on a baking sheet. Roast for 30-40 minutes, or until tender.
2. **Cook Filling:** While squash roasts, heat olive oil in a skillet. Cook ground turkey, breaking it up, until browned. Add onion and garlic, cook until softened. Stir in quinoa, cranberries, walnuts, sage, salt, and pepper.
3. **Stuff & Bake:** Flip roasted squash halves. Fill with the turkey-quinoa mixture, mounding slightly. Sprinkle with feta cheese (if using). Bake for 10-15 minutes more, until heated through.

Prep Time: 15 minutes **Cook Time:** 45-55 minutes

Nutritional Info (approx. per stuffed half):
- Calories: 450, Sodium: 350mg (without feta), Potassium: 800mg, Fiber: 10g, Protein: 30g

Tips:
- Substitute ground turkey with another lean protein like ground chicken or crumbled tofu.
- Add other POTS-friendly chopped vegetables to the filling, like bell peppers, mushrooms, or spinach.
- Use a different type of dried fruit like chopped apricots or cherries.

Chapter 5: Snacks, Sips, and Smart Choices

Savory Snacks

Salty Trail Mix

- **POTS Power:** This mix is loaded with salty nuts (almonds, pistachios, peanuts), pumpkin seeds, and even a bit of dried seaweed (if tolerated) for an extra mineral boost.
- **Snack Time Delight:** A super satisfying mix, perfect for on-the-go snacking or when you crave something crunchy and salty.

Ingredients:

- 1/2 cup salted almonds
- 1/2 cup salted pistachios
- 1/2 cup salted peanuts
- 1/4 cup roasted pumpkin seeds
- 2 tablespoons crumbled dried seaweed flakes (optional, but adds an extra salty kick)
- 1/4 cup pretzels (for an extra dose of carbs)

Instructions:

1. **Combine:** Simply toss all ingredients together in a bowl or container. Enjoy!

Prep Time: 5 minutes

Nutritional Info (approx. per 1/4 cup serving):

- Calories: 200, Sodium: 300mg, Potassium: 300mg, Fiber: 5g, Protein: 10g

Tips:

- Customize with your favorite salty nuts and seeds.
- Add a touch of spice with a pinch of cayenne pepper or smoked paprika.
- Store in an airtight container for grab-and-go snacking.

Pickle Roll-Ups

- **POTS Power:** Cream cheese offers a touch of creaminess, deli meat provides protein, and pickles deliver that salty, vinegary goodness.
- **Snack Time Delight:** A tangy and satisfying snack that's quick and easy to make.

Ingredients:

- 4 thin slices deli ham or salami
- 2 ounces cream cheese, softened
- 4 dill pickle spears

Instructions:

1. **Spread:** Spread a thin layer of cream cheese onto each slice of deli meat.
2. **Roll:** Place a pickle spear at one end of the meat slice and roll it up. Slice roll-ups into bite-sized pieces.

Prep Time: 5 minutes

Nutritional Info (approx. per 2 roll-ups):

- Calories: 150, Sodium: 450mg, Potassium: 150mg, Fat: 12g, Protein: 8g

Tips:

- Use lower-sodium deli meat and pickles if possible.
- Experiment with different deli meats like turkey or roast beef.
- Add a tiny dollop of Dijon mustard to the center of the cream cheese before rolling for an extra flavor kick.

Mini Cheese & Olive Skewers

- **POTS Power:** Cheese offers saltiness and protein, while olives provide healthy fats and additional salty flavor.
- **Snack Time Delight:** A simple yet elegant snack, perfect for a quick bite or even as a fun appetizer.

Ingredients:

- 4 ounces cheddar or mozzarella cheese, cut into small cubes
- 8 green or black olives
- Toothpicks

Instructions:

1. **Assemble:** Thread a cheese cube and an olive onto each toothpick, alternating as desired.

Prep Time: 5 minutes

Nutritional Info (approx. per 2 skewers):

- Calories: 100, Sodium: 350mg, Potassium: 100mg, Fat: 8g, Protein: 6g

Tips:

- Use a variety of cheeses like Gouda, Swiss, or pepper jack.
- Add a small cherry tomato to each skewer for a pop of color.

- Dining Out and Special Occasions (Tips for navigating menus and making POTS-friendly choices)

Crunchy Corned Beef Bites

- **POTS Power:** Leftover corned beef offers a salty protein boost, while Dijon mustard and mayonnaise add satisfying creaminess and flavor.
- **Snack Time Delight:** A simple and tasty way to repurpose leftovers and get a savory, satisfying snack. Serve with whole-grain crackers or cucumber slices for scooping.

Ingredients:

- 1 cup shredded leftover corned beef
- 1 tablespoon Dijon mustard
- 2 tablespoons mayonnaise
- Whole-grain crackers or cucumber slices for serving

Instructions:

1. **Mix:** In a bowl, combine corned beef with Dijon mustard and mayonnaise. Mix until well combined.
2. **Serve:** Serve with whole-grain crackers or cucumber slices.

Prep Time: 5 minutes

Nutritional Info (approx. per 1/4 cup serving):

- Calories: 180, Sodium: 350mg, Potassium: 200mg, Fat: 12g, Protein: 10g

Tips:

- If you don't have leftover corned beef, use canned corned beef hash.
- Adjust the amount of mustard or mayonnaise to your liking.
- Add a pinch of black pepper for extra flavor.

Savory Yogurt Dip

- **POTS Power:** Greek yogurt provides protein and a creamy base, while miso paste adds a savory, salty depth of flavor. Chives and pepper offer a freshness that balances the richness.
- **Snack Time Delight:** A unique and flavorful dip that's perfect for pairing with crunchy vegetables.

Ingredients:
- 1/2 cup plain Greek yogurt
- 1 teaspoon miso paste (start with less if unsure, taste, and add more if desired)
- 2 tablespoons chopped chives
- Pinch of black pepper
- Vegetable sticks (carrots, celery, cucumbers, bell peppers) for dipping

Instructions:
1. **Mix:** Combine yogurt, miso paste, chives, and black pepper in a bowl. Mix well.
2. **Serve:** Serve with your favorite vegetable dippers.

Prep Time: 5 minutes

Nutritional Info (approx. per 2 tablespoons of dip):
- Calories: 30, Sodium: 100mg, Potassium: 100mg, Fat: 1g, Protein: 4g

Tips:
- Use a low-sodium miso paste if possible.
- Experiment with different herbs like fresh dill or parsley.
- For extra richness, stir in a dollop of sour cream.

Hard-Boiled Eggs with Everything Seasoning

- **POTS Power:** Eggs offer protein and a good dose of natural sodium. "Everything bagel" seasoning adds a burst of savory flavor with a satisfying salty kick.
- **Snack Time Delight:** A classic snack that's quick, easy, and boosted with bold flavor.

Ingredients:

- 2 hard-boiled eggs, peeled and halved
- 1 teaspoon "everything bagel" seasoning

Instructions:

1. **Season:** Sprinkle "everything bagel" seasoning generously over the cut sides of the hard-boiled eggs.

Prep Time: 5 minutes

Nutritional Info (approx. per 1 egg):

- Calories: 80, Sodium: 150mg, Potassium: 70mg, Fat: 6g, Protein: 6g

Tips:

- Make a larger batch of hard-boiled eggs and keep them in the fridge for easy snacking throughout the week.
- If you can't find "everything bagel" seasoning, make your own blend with sesame seeds, poppy seeds, dried onion flakes, dried garlic flakes, and a pinch of salt.

Spicy Roasted Chickpeas

- **POTS Power:** Chickpeas are a good source of protein and fiber, while the spices add flavor and warmth.
- **Snack Time Delight:** A crunchy, satisfying, and portable snack option packed with flavor.

Ingredients:

- 1 (15-ounce) can chickpeas, rinsed and drained
- 1 tablespoon olive oil
- 1/2 teaspoon smoked paprika
- 1/4 teaspoon cumin
- Pinch of cayenne pepper
- Salt to taste.

Instructions:

1. **Prep & Season:** Pat chickpeas dry with a paper towel. Toss with olive oil, paprika, cumin, cayenne, and salt.
2. **Roast:** Spread chickpeas on baking sheet. Roast at 400°F (200°C) for 20-25 minutes, or until golden and crispy.

Prep Time: 5 minutes **Cook Time:** 20-25 minutes

Nutritional Info (approx. per 1/2 cup serving):

- Calories: 150, Sodium: 100mg, Potassium: 200mg, Fiber: 6g, Protein: 8g

Tips:

- Experiment with different spice blends (curry powder, chili powder, etc.).
- Add a squeeze of lemon juice after roasting for a touch of brightness.

Hydrating & Refreshing
Fruit & Veggie Skewers

- **POTS Power:** Melon (like watermelon and honeydew) provides hydration and electrolytes, cucumbers offer additional hydration, and grapes contain antioxidants.
- **Snack Time Delight:** Colorful, refreshing, and naturally sweet – perfect for a light and healthy snack.

Ingredients:

- Chunks of watermelon
- Chunks of honeydew melon
- Cucumber slices
- Grapes

Instructions:

1. **Assemble:** Thread melon chunks, cucumber slices, and grapes onto skewers, alternating for a colorful presentation.

Prep Time: 5-10 minutes

Nutritional Info (approx. per skewer with 4-5 pieces of fruit):

- Calories: 50, Sodium: 20mg, Potassium: 200mg, Fiber: 2g, Vitamin C: 15% DV

Tips:

- Use other hydrating fruits like strawberries, blueberries, or pineapple chunks.
- For extra sweetness, drizzle skewers with a touch of honey.

Chia Seed Pudding

- **POTS Power:** Chia seeds absorb liquid and create a creamy pudding. They offer fiber, healthy fats, and a boost of various nutrients. Almond milk provides hydration, and a touch of maple syrup and vanilla adds sweetness.
- **Snack Time Delight:** This satisfying snack takes minutes to prepare but sets in the fridge for a grab-and-go treat.

Ingredients
- 1/4 cup chia seeds
- 1 cup unsweetened almond milk
- 1 tablespoon maple syrup
- 1/4 teaspoon vanilla extract

Instructions:
1. **Combine:** In a jar or container, whisk together chia seeds, almond milk, maple syrup, and vanilla extract.
2. **Chill & Set:** Refrigerate for at least 2 hours, or preferably overnight, until pudding thickens.
3. **Enjoy:** Top with berries, chopped nuts, or a sprinkle of granola for extra crunch (optional).

Prep Time: 5 minutes (plus setting time in the fridge)

Nutritional Info (approx. per serving):
- Calories: 180, Sodium: 80mg, Potassium: 200mg, Fiber: 8g, Protein: 6g

Tips:
- Substitute with your preferred plant-based milk.
- Adjust the amount of maple syrup for desired sweetness.
- Play with flavors: add cocoa powder, cinnamon, or a pinch of cardamom.

Frozen Grapes

- **POTS Power:** Grapes are high in water content, providing hydration and a touch of natural sweetness. Freezing them adds a refreshing, icy element.
- **Snack Time Delight:** The simplest of snacks! Perfect for those hot days when you need a quick, cooling treat.

Ingredients:

- 1 cup grapes (green or red)

Instructions:

1. **Wash & Freeze:** Wash grapes and pat dry. Spread on a baking sheet and freeze for at least 2 hours, or until solid.
2. **Enjoy:** Pop them straight from the freezer for a refreshing snack.

Prep Time: 5 minutes (plus freezing time)

Nutritional Info (approx. per 1/2 cup):

- Calories: 50, Sodium: 5mg, Potassium: 150mg, Fiber: 1g, Vitamin C: 5% DV

Tips:

- Try freezing other fruits like berries or melon chunks.
- Frozen grapes make a fun addition to water or sparkling water.

Banana "Nice Cream"

- **POTS Power:** Bananas are rich in potassium and offer natural sweetness. Blended frozen, they create a creamy, ice-cream-like treat.
- **Snack Time Delight:** A healthy and satisfying way to enjoy a sweet and cool dessert-like snack.

Ingredients:
- 2 frozen bananas, cut into chunks
- 1/4 cup milk (almond milk, soy milk, etc., or a bit more if needed)
- Optional: 1 tablespoon cocoa powder (for chocolate flavor)

Instructions:
1. **Blend:** Add frozen bananas and milk to a blender or food processor. Blend until smooth and creamy, scraping down sides as needed. For chocolate flavor, add cocoa powder and blend.
2. **Serve:** Enjoy immediately for a soft-serve consistency, or freeze for a firmer ice cream texture.

Prep Time: 5 minutes

Nutritional Info (approx. per serving, without cocoa):
- Calories: 200, Sodium: 30mg, Potassium: 800mg, Fiber: 6g

Tips:
- Use very ripe bananas for the best sweetness and texture.
- Add other flavorings like a pinch of cinnamon, vanilla extract, or a spoonful of peanut butter.
- Top with chopped nuts, fresh berries, or a drizzle of honey for extra flavor and texture.

Avocado Smoothie

- **POTS Power:** Avocado offers healthy fats and potassium, spinach provides electrolytes and nutrients, banana adds sweetness and potassium, and almond milk boosts hydration.
- **Snack Time Delight:** This creamy and satisfying smoothie is packed with nutrients and makes a refreshing on-the-go snack.

Ingredients:
- 1/2 avocado, pitted and peeled
- 1 cup packed baby spinach
- 1 frozen banana, cut into chunks
- 1 cup unsweetened almond milk
- Squeeze of lime juice

Instructions:
1. **Blend:** Combine all ingredients in a blender and blend until completely smooth.
2. **Enjoy:** Pour into a glass and enjoy immediately.

Prep Time: 5 minutes

Nutritional Info (approx. per serving):
- Calories: 250, Sodium: 100mg, Potassium: 900mg, Fiber: 10g, Protein: 8g

Tips:
- Add a scoop of your favorite protein powder for an extra boost.
- Use other plant-based milk options like soy milk or oat milk.
- For a sweeter smoothie, add a tablespoon of honey or maple syrup.

Electrolyte Popsicles

- **POTS Power:** Watermelon and cucumber provide hydration, a small amount of salt helps retain fluids, and a squeeze of lime adds a refreshing citrus boost.
- **Snack Time Delight:** These homemade popsicles are a fun and delicious way to get extra hydration and electrolytes – perfect for a hot day.

Ingredients:

- 2 cups cubed watermelon
- 1/2 cup diced cucumber
- Pinch of salt
- Squeeze of lime juice

Instructions:

1. **Blend:** Combine watermelon, cucumber, salt, and lime juice in a blender. Blend until smooth.
2. **Freeze:** Pour mixture into popsicle molds and freeze for at least 4 hours or until solid.

Prep Time: 10 minutes (plus freezing time)

Nutritional Info (approx. per popsicle):

- Calories: 30, Sodium: 50mg, Potassium: 150mg, Fiber: 1g

Tips:

- Get creative with the shapes of your popsicle molds!
- Add other POTS-friendly fruits like berries or melon chunks.

Fruit-Infused Water

- **POTS Power:** Water is the ultimate hydrator, and the addition of fruit and herbs provides subtle flavor and a touch of natural sweetness.
- **Snack Time Delight:** A refreshing and healthy alternative to sugary drinks or plain water.

Ingredients:
- Pitcher of cold water
- Sliced cucumbers and/or citrus fruits (lemons, limes, oranges)
- Fresh berries (strawberries, blueberries, raspberries)
- Fresh herbs (mint, basil)

Instructions:
1. **Infuse:** Add sliced cucumbers, citrus fruits, berries, and herbs to a pitcher of cold water. Give it a gentle muddle with a spoon to release some of the juices.
2. **Chill:** Refrigerate for at least 2 hours, or preferably overnight, to allow flavors to infuse.
3. **Enjoy:** Pour over ice and enjoy!

Prep Time: 5 minutes (plus infusing time)

Tips:
- Get creative with your flavor combinations! Experiment with different fruits, herbs, and even spices like ginger.
- The longer you infuse, the stronger the flavor will be.
- Refill the pitcher with fresh water throughout the day and keep adding new fruit and herbs as needed.

Herbal Iced Tea

- **POTS Power:** Herbal teas are naturally caffeine-free and offer various health benefits depending on the herbs used.
- **Snack Time Delight:** A flavorful and refreshing alternative to water, especially when served iced.

Ingredients:
- 4 cups water
- 2-3 tablespoons loose leaf herbal tea (chamomile, peppermint, hibiscus, or your favorite blend)
- Lemon wedges (optional)
- Honey or maple syrup to taste (optional)

Instructions:
1. **Brew:** Bring water to a boil. Remove from heat and add herbal tea. Allow to steep for 5-10 minutes (depending on desired strength).
2. **Strain & Chill:** Strain tea into a pitcher. Refrigerate until fully chilled.
3. **Serve:** Pour over ice and add a squeeze of lemon or a touch of sweetener if desired.

Prep Time: 5 minutes (plus brewing and chilling time)

Tips:
- Explore different herbal tea blends. Chamomile is calming, peppermint promotes digestion, and hibiscus has a tart, fruity flavor.
- Sweeten to your liking. If adding honey, do so once the tea has cooled to preserve its beneficial properties.

Chapter 6: Living Well with POTS

Beyond the Plate: Lifestyle Factors

While a POTS-friendly diet is a crucial foundation, true success in managing POTS involves a holistic approach. Here's where lifestyle factors can make a huge difference:

Exercise:

1. **The Challenge:** Exercise can be a double-edged sword for those with POTS. It's essential for long-term health but finding the right type and intensity is key, as overexertion can worsen symptoms.
2. **Gentle Starts:** Begin with low-impact activities like walking, swimming, or recumbent biking for short durations.
3. **Gradual Progression:** Slowly increase the intensity and duration of exercise as tolerated.
4. **Focus on Consistency:** Aim for regular activity rather than occasional strenuous workouts.

5. **Listen to Your Body:** Pay extreme attention to how your body reacts during and after exercise. Rest when needed and adjust accordingly.

Stress Management:

1. **The Impact:** Stress can significantly exacerbate POTS symptoms.
2. **Stress-Busting Techniques:** Practice mindfulness, meditation, deep breathing exercises, yoga, or gentle stretching. These techniques lower stress hormones and promote relaxation.
3. **Therapy:** Consider cognitive behavioral therapy (CBT) to develop coping skills and change thought patterns that worsen stress.
4. **Enjoyable Activities:** Make time for hobbies and activities that bring you joy and reduce stress.

Sleep Tips:

1. **The Need:** Sufficient, quality sleep is vital for POTS management but can be elusive.
2. **Sleep Hygiene:** Create a calming bedtime routine, maintain regular sleep hours, and ensure your bedroom is dark, quiet, and cool.
3. **Avoid Naps:** If nighttime sleep is difficult, try to resist naps that disrupt the sleep-wake cycle.

4. **Talk to Your Doctor:** Discuss medications or sleep aids if poor sleep persists.

The Importance of Individualization

POTS is a complex condition that affects people differently. It is essential to remember that there is no single approach that works for everyone.

- **Working with a Dietician/Healthcare Provider:** A registered dietician specializing in POTS can personalize your dietary needs. Partner with your doctor to develop an overall treatment plan that may include exercise guidance, medication, and other therapies.
- **Be Patient & Persistent:** Finding the right mix of diet, exercise, stress management, and sleep habits takes time and experimentation.
- **Seek Support:** Connect with POTS support groups online or in your community for encouragement and shared experiences.

Success Story: Alex's Journey

Alex had struggled with POTS for years. The dizziness, fatigue, and heart palpitations left them feeling overwhelmed and discouraged. After being diagnosed, they started researching POTS-friendly diets but felt lost amidst the confusing information.

Discovering The cookbook was a turning point for Alex. The clear explanations and delicious recipes made eating for POTS feel doable and even enjoyable. They learned how to boost salt intake with satisfying snacks, stay hydrated with flavorful drinks, and ensure they were getting essential nutrients.

The changes weren't immediate, but slowly and steadily, Alex started feeling better. They had more energy, and their flare-ups became less frequent. They even found a gentle yoga class that helped them build strength and manage stress.

Alex's story reminds us that managing POTS is a marathon, not a sprint. With the right tools, support, and a willingness to experiment, it's absolutely possible to improve your quality of life.

THANK YOU!!!

Your Feedback Matters!

My hope is that this cookbook has been a helpful resource on your POTS journey. I'd love to hear how it's helped you and how it can be even better!

Please Leave a Review

The best way to share your experience is to leave a review. Your honest feedback will help others with POTS discover this resource and allow me to improve it for the future. Here's what you can share:

- **Recipe Successes:** Which recipes were your favorites?

- **Your Adaptations:** How did you make the recipes work even better for you?
- **Everyday Tips:** Did the cookbook inspire you with helpful lifestyle tips?
- **Your Story:** Has this cookbook made a difference in your life?

Your feedback is invaluable. It will help me, and future readers, continue to learn and improve resources for navigating POTS with confidence and deliciousness!

Appendix

7-day meal plan

POTS SYNDROME WEEKLY MEAL TRACKER

	BREAKFAST	LUNCH	DINNER	SNACKS &
MON	Avocado & Everything Oats	Coconut Curry Butternut Squash Soup	One-Pan Roasted Chicken & Veggies	Fruit & Veggie Skewers, Hard-boiled Egg with Everything Seasoning WATER ■ ■ ■ ■ ■ ■ ■ ■
TUE	Tropical Overnight Oats	Mediterranean Quinoa Salad	Lentil & Mushroom "Shepherd's Pie"	Salty Trail Mix, Mini Cheese & Olive Skewers WATER ■ ■ ■ ■ ■ ■ ■ ■
WED	Savory Spinach & Egg Scramble Oats	Hearty Minestrone Soup	Tuna Salad Lettuce Wraps	Chia Seed Pudding, Spicy Roasted Chickpeas WATER ■ ■ ■ ■ ■ ■
THU	Pumpkin Spice Power Oats	Chicken & Veggie Stuffed Peppers	Shrimp Scampi with Zucchini Noodles	Pickle Roll-Ups, Frozen Grapes WATER ■ ■ ■ ■ ■ ■
FRI	"PB&B" Bowl	Spicy Chicken & Corn Chowder	Summer Veggie Frittata	Banana "Nice Cream", Savory Yogurt Dip WATER ■ ■ ■ ■ ■
SAT	Green Powerhouse Smoothie	Southwest Black Bean & Avocado Salad	Salmon & Roasted Veggie Bowls	Avocado Smoothie, Crunchy Corned Beef Bites WATER ■ ■ ■ ■ ■ ■ ■
SUN	Avocado Toast Upgrade	Asian Noodle Salad	Chicken Pot Pie with Sweet Potato Crust	Electrolyte Popsicles, Fruit-Infused Water WATER ■ ■ ■ ■ ■ ■

Important Notes:

- **Hydration:** Drink plenty of water throughout the day, especially between meals. Consider adding electrolyte drinks or making your own as needed.
- **Salt:** This plan incorporates many salty options but adjust based on your individual needs. Listen to your body and your healthcare provider!
- **Snacks:** Include snacks as needed to prevent blood sugar dips and help manage POTS symptoms.
- **Portions:** Pay attention to portion sizes and how your body feels. You might need smaller, more frequent meals or larger portions depending on your individual needs.
- **Variety:** This is just one possible week! Aim for variety to ensure you're getting a wide range of nutrients. Swap in other options from the list as you like.

Food Conversion Charts (Sodium content, etc.)

What are Food Conversion Charts?

Food conversion charts are resources that provide various measurements or nutrient information about common foods. Here are the main types relevant to POTS:

- **Sodium Conversion Charts:** These focus specifically on the sodium content of foods. They often list foods in common serving sizes (e.g., 1 cup, 1 slice, 1 medium fruit) along with the corresponding amount of sodium in milligrams (mg).

- **Nutrient Composition Databases:** More comprehensive databases that include not just sodium, but also other nutrients like potassium, carbohydrates, protein, etc. Popular examples include the USDA FoodData Central database (https://fdc.nal.usda.gov/).

Why Use Them for POTS Management?

- **Track Sodium Intake:** Those with POTS often need higher sodium intake. Conversion charts help you make informed food choices and track your daily sodium intake to ensure you're hitting your targets.
- **Identify High-Sodium Foods:** Charts let you quickly compare similar foods, revealing ones surprisingly high in sodium. This empowers you to make swaps for lower sodium versions.
- **Estimate Sodium in Recipes:** When cooking for yourself, use charts to estimate the total sodium content of your meals, helping you make necessary adjustments.

How to Use Food Conversion Charts

1. **Find Reliable Charts:** Here are some good sources:

    - **Websites:** The American Heart Association , Centers for Disease Control and Prevention (CDC), and reputable health organizations often have downloadable charts.
    - **Apps:** Apps like "MyFitnessPal" and "Lose It!" have food databases that include sodium information.
    - **Product Labels:** While not as comprehensive as dedicated charts, food labels always list sodium per serving.

2. **Understand Serving Sizes:** Pay close attention to the serving sizes listed on the chart. Is it realistic for how much you typically eat? For example, one slice of bread might have 200mg sodium, but if you eat two, that's 400mg.

3. **Compare Foods:** Use the chart to compare your usual choices. For example, you might be surprised how much more sodium is in canned soup vs. homemade.

4. **Track Your Intake:** If your doctor has given you a sodium goal, track your intake throughout the day using information from the charts.

Important Notes:

- **Food Processing Matters:** The same type of food can vary in sodium content depending on the brand and how it's processed. Fresh, whole foods are usually lower in sodium than heavily processed versions.
- **Charts are Estimates:** Sodium content can fluctuate even within the same brand; consider charts a helpful guide, not an absolute measure.
- **It's Not Just About Salt:** Many processed foods contain "hidden" sodium. Read ingredient lists carefully for sources of sodium like monosodium glutamate (MSG), baking soda, and sodium phosphates.

Example: Let's say you're making chili, here's how to use a chart:

1. **Ingredients:** Look up the sodium content per serving for each ingredient (canned beans, tomatoes, ground beef, etc.)
2. **Calculate:** Multiply the sodium per serving by the number of servings of that ingredient you're using. Do this for each ingredient.
3. **Add It Up:** Add the sodium totals from each ingredient to estimate the total sodium for the whole batch of chili.
4. **Divide:** Divide the total sodium content by the number of servings your recipe makes for the per-serving estimate.

28 DAYS MEAL PLANNER TEMPLATE & SHOPPING LIST

WEEK 1
POTS SYNDROME WEEKLY MEAL TRACKER

	BREAKFAST	LUNCH	DINNER	SNACKS &
MON				WATER ☐☐☐☐☐☐☐☐
TUE				WATER ☐☐☐☐☐☐☐☐
WED				WATER ☐☐☐☐☐☐☐☐
THU				WATER ☐☐☐☐☐☐☐☐
FRI				WATER ☐☐☐☐☐☐☐☐
SAT				WATER ☐☐☐☐☐☐☐☐
SUN				WATER ☐☐☐☐☐☐☐☐

WEEKLY SHOPPING LIST

DATE: _____

FRUITS AND VEGETABLES	DAIRY AND EGGS	MEAT AND POULTRY

SEAFOOD	PANTRY STAPLES	BREADS AND GRAINS

BEVERAGES	SNACKS AND SWEETS	HOUSEHOLD ITEMS

WEEK 2
POTS SYNDROME WEEKLY MEAL TRACKER

	BREAKFAST	LUNCH	DINNER	SNACKS &
MON				WATER ☐☐☐☐☐☐☐☐
TUE				WATER ☐☐☐☐☐☐☐☐
WED				WATER ☐☐☐☐☐☐☐☐
THU				WATER ☐☐☐☐☐☐☐☐
FRI				WATER ☐☐☐☐☐☐☐☐
SAT				WATER ☐☐☐☐☐☐☐☐
SUN				WATER ☐☐☐☐☐☐☐☐

WEEKLY SHOPPING LIST

DATE: _____

FRUITS AND VEGETABLES	DAIRY AND EGGS	MEAT AND POULTRY

SEAFOOD	PANTRY STAPLES	BREADS AND GRAINS

BEVERAGES	SNACKS AND SWEETS	HOUSEHOLD ITEMS

WEEK 3
POTS SYNDROME WEEKLY MEAL TRACKER

	BREAKFAST	LUNCH	DINNER	SNACKS &
MON				WATER ☐☐☐☐☐☐☐
TUE				WATER ☐☐☐☐☐☐☐
WED				WATER ☐☐☐☐☐☐☐
THU				WATER ☐☐☐☐☐☐☐
FRI				WATER ☐☐☐☐☐☐☐
SAT				WATER ☐☐☐☐☐☐☐
SUN				WATER ☐☐☐☐☐☐☐

WEEKLY SHOPPING LIST

DATE: _____

FRUITS AND VEGETABLES	DAIRY AND EGGS	MEAT AND POULTRY

SEAFOOD	PANTRY STAPLES	BREADS AND GRAINS

BEVERAGES	SNACKS AND SWEETS	HOUSEHOLD ITEMS

Avery Stoneheart

WEEK 4

POTS SYNDROME WEEKLY MEAL TRACKER

	BREAKFAST	LUNCH	DINNER	SNACKS &
MON				WATER ☐☐☐☐☐☐☐
TUE				WATER ☐☐☐☐☐☐☐
WED				WATER ☐☐☐☐☐☐☐
THU				WATER ☐☐☐☐☐☐☐
FRI				WATER ☐☐☐☐☐☐☐
SAT				WATER ☐☐☐☐☐☐☐
SUN				WATER ☐☐☐☐☐☐☐

WEEKLY SHOPPING LIST

DATE: _____

FRUITS AND VEGETABLES	DAIRY AND EGGS	MEAT AND POULTRY

SEAFOOD	PANTRY STAPLES	BREADS AND GRAINS

BEVERAGES	SNACKS AND SWEETS	HOUSEHOLD ITEMS

www.ingramcontent.com/pod-product-compliance
Lightning Source LLC
Chambersburg PA
CBHW050300230526
45471CB00005B/1964